SpringerBriefs in
Specialty Topics in Behavioral Medicine

Series Editor
Joost Dekker

For further volumes:
http://www.springer.com/series/11956

Joost Dekker

Editor

Exercise and Physical Functioning in Osteoarthritis

Medical, Neuromuscular and Behavioral Perspectives

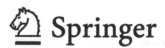
Springer

Editor
Joost Dekker
Department of Rehabilitation Medicine
and Department of Psychiatry
VU University Medical Center
Amsterdam, The Netherlands

ISBN 978-1-4614-7214-8   ISBN 978-1-4614-7215-5 (eBook)
DOI 10.1007/978-1-4614-7215-5
Springer New York Heidelberg Dordrecht London

Library of Congress Control Number: 2013943272

Printed on acid-free paper

Springer is part of Springer Science+Business Media (www.springer.com)

Contents

Contributors

Mariëtte de Rooij Amsterdam Rehabilitation Research Center | Reade, Amsterdam, The Netherlands

Joost Dekker Department of Rehabilitation Medicine, VU University Medical Center, Amsterdam, The Netherlands

Department of Psychiatry, VU University Medical Center, Amsterdam, The Netherlands

Martijn Gerritsen Department of Rheumatology | Reade, Amsterdam, The Netherlands

Jasmijn F.M. Holla Amsterdam Rehabilitation Research Center | Reade, Amsterdam, The Netherlands

Jesper Knoop Amsterdam Rehabilitation Research Center | Reade, Amsterdam, The Netherlands

Willem F. Lems Department of Rheumatology, VU University Medical Center, Amsterdam, The Netherlands

Wilfred Peter Amsterdam Rehabilitation Research Center | Reade, Amsterdam, The Netherlands

Martijn Pisters Clinical Health Sciences, University Medical Center Utrecht, Utrecht, The Netherlands

Leo D. Roorda Amsterdam Rehabilitation Research Center | Reade, Amsterdam, The Netherlands

Diana C. Sanchez-Ramirez Faculty of Human Movement Sciences, VU University, Amsterdam, The Netherlands

Martijn P.M. Steultjens School of Health and Life Sciences, Institute for Applied Health Research, Glasgow Caledonian University, Glasgow, Lanarkshire, UK

Martin van der Esch Amsterdam Rehabilitation Research Center | Reade, Amsterdam, The Netherlands

Marike van der Leeden Amsterdam Rehabilitation Research Center | Reade, Amsterdam, The Netherlands

Cindy Veenhof Netherlands Institute for Health Services Research (NIVEL), Utrecht, The Netherlands

Ramon E. Voorneman Department of Rheumatology | Reade, Amsterdam, The Netherlands

Chapter 1
Introduction

Joost Dekker

Osteoarthritis (OA) is the major cause of pain and activity limitations among the elderly [1]. Recent research has shown that behavioral factors, neuromuscular factors, and medical factors predict pain and activity limitations in OA. Examples include lack of physical activity, muscle weakness, and comorbidity, respectively.

Exercise therapy is among the dominant interventions in OA. Exercise therapy has been shown to effectively reduce pain and activity limitations in OA. Recently, innovative exercise interventions have been developed. These innovative approaches toward exercise target neuromuscular and behavioral factors and are tailored to the patient's medical condition.

Research in this field has been published as separate empirical papers, with limited background information. This field is in need of an integrative contextual review, summarizing the separate papers and putting the empirical research into theoretical perspective. The objectives of this book on OA of the knee or hip are:

1. To summarize knowledge on the epidemiology, pathogenesis, clinical aspects, and therapeutic options.
2. To review recent research on behavioral and neuromuscular factors in functional decline, with a special emphasis on explanatory mechanisms.
3. To review innovative approaches toward exercise therapy, derived from research on behavioral, neuromuscular, and medical factors.

The remainder of this chapter provides a short introduction to these issues.

J. Dekker (✉)
Department of Rehabilitation Medicine, VU University Medical Center, PO Box 7057, 1007 MB Amsterdam, The Netherlands

Department of Psychiatry, VU University Medical Center, Amsterdam, The Netherlands
e-mail: j.dekker@vumc.nl

J. Dekker (ed.), *Exercise and Physical Functioning in Osteoarthritis: Medical, Neuromuscular and Behavioral Perspectives*, Springer Briefs in Specialty Topics in Behavioral Medicine, DOI 10.1007/978-1-4614-7215-5_1, © The Author(s) 2014

Osteoarthritis of the Knee or Hip

Osteoarthritis (OA) is a major public health issue. In a study in the USA, the prevalence of symptomatic OA of the knee or hip was estimated as 16.7 % and 9.2 %, respectively [2]. In the European region OA is among the ten most disabling conditions [1]. Because of the aging population and because of the increasing prevalence of overweight, a dramatic increase in the prevalence of OA and its related pain and activity limitations is expected [3]. OA frequently affects the knee and the hip; other joints, such as the hand, are also frequently involved. The *first objective* of this book is to summarize knowledge on epidemiology, pathogenesis, clinical aspects, and therapeutic options in OA of the knee or hip.

Functional Decline in Osteoarthritis of the Knee or Hip

Pain is a major symptom of OA. Subjects with OA of the knee or hip experience a continuous pain: they describe this as dull or aching pain. This is interspersed with short episodes of unpredictable and intense pain [4]. Other impairments and symptoms observed in subjects with OA include muscle weakness, stiffness, reduced range of motion of the joints, and instability or buckling of the knee joint.

OA related impairments and symptoms cause activity limitations such as limitations in walking, climbing stairs, sitting down, rising up, bending down, and lifting. Activity limitations may translate into restrictions in social participation; examples of restrictions in participation include problems with housekeeping, shopping, travelling, sports, and work.

Activity limitations develop more progressively in subjects with OA than in subjects without OA; subjects who have osteoarthritis at middle age are more likely to develop persistent activity limitations such as difficulty with mobility or ADL function in the next 10 years [5]. However, functional decline is a slow process; at group level, worsening of pain and activity limitations becomes evident only after 3 or more years of follow-up [6].

The course of activity limitations in OA of the knee or hip is highly individual and variable: functioning has been found to improve in some patients, to remain stable in others, and to gradually worsen in still others [7, 8]. Because of this variability, identification of risk factors for functional decline is of utmost importance. Knowledge on risk factors can be used to inform patients on the likely course of their condition. Knowledge on risk factors also contributes to the understanding of mechanisms and processes, which cause functional decline. A better understanding of these mechanisms and processes contributes to the development of therapeutic and preventive interventions, aiming at recovery of functioning or prevention of functional decline, respectively.

Risk Factors and Explanatory Mechanisms

A wide range of risk factors for functional decline has been identified: risk factors range from comorbid conditions such as diabetes and cardiovascular conditions, impairments such as pain and muscle weakness, to behavioral factors such as lack of physical activity, and psychological factors such as anxiety and depression [7].

A risk factor provides information on the prognosis: subjects with a high-risk profile are likely to show functional decline. In itself, a risk factor does not explain how functional decline comes about; a risk factor predicts but does not explain functional decline. On the other hand, the risk factor can be integrated into an explanatory model or theory on functional decline; in that case, knowledge on the risk factor does contribute to our understanding of the mechanism of functional decline.

Avoidance of Activity

Avoidance of activity is an explanation for functional decline in OA of the knee, and possibly also OA of the hip. According to this explanation, pain may cause subjects to avoid activity. In OA, pain is frequently related to activities such as walking; avoidance of these activities reduces pain. In the short term, this is beneficial; avoidance of activity causes less pain. In the long term, however, avoidance of activity is contributing to the development of activity limitations. Physical activity and exercise are required to maintain muscles strength. Avoidance of activity causes muscle weakness and muscle weakness is one of the most important causes of activity limitations. In summary, avoidance of pain-related activity is hypothesized to cause muscle weakness, and thereby activity limitations. This theory is illustrated in Fig. 1.1.

Psychological distress, such as an anxious and depressive mood, is a risk factor for activity limitations in OA. Psychological distress is thought to enhance the tendency to avoid activity, resulting in muscle weakness and activity limitations (see Fig. 1.1). Thus, avoidance of activity is hypothesized to explain how psychological distress affects activity limitations.

Neuromuscular Factors

Muscle weakness is a crucial factor in the behavioral explanation of functional decline in OA. Muscle weakness is thought to have a *direct* impact on the activity limitations; muscle strength is required for the adequate performance of activities. Muscle weakness may also have an *indirect* impact on the performance of activities via instability of the knee joint. Strong muscles contribute to the ability of the knee

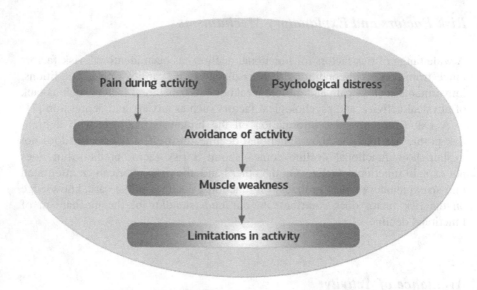

Fig. 1.1 Behavioral explanation of activity limitations: avoidance of activity

joint to maintain a position or to control movements under differing external loads. Muscle weakness is thought to cause instability of the knee, and thereby limitations in activity.

Other neuromuscular factors are involved in stabilizing the knee as well. This applies in particular to proprioception—the sense of joint motion and position. Good proprioceptive acuity is required for the performance of activities, in addition to muscle strength. Conversely, poor proprioception is hypothesized to strengthen the impact of muscle weakness on activity limitations: decreased proprioceptive acuity aggravates the impact of muscle weakness on activity limitations. This is illustrated in Fig. 1.2.

Laxity of the knee joint refers to the passive range of motion in the frontal plane. Laxity is hypothesized to cause instability of the knee, and thereby activity limitations. In a lax knee, stability can be achieved by more muscle strength; stronger muscles may compensate laxity. Conversely, laxity may aggravate the impact of muscle weakness on activity limitations; muscle weakness in combination with laxity has an even stronger impact on activity limitations. The combined impact of laxity and muscle weakness on activity limitations is illustrated in Fig. 1.2.

Knee varus–valgus motion is the movement of the knee in the frontal plane during walking. High varus–valgus motion is hypothesized to contribute to instability of the knee. Muscle strength may compensate varus–valgus motion. This implies that patients with high varus–valgus motion need more muscle strength to perform activities. Conversely, high varus–valgus motion is hypothesized to aggravate the impact of muscle weakness on activity limitations as illustrated in Fig. 1.2.

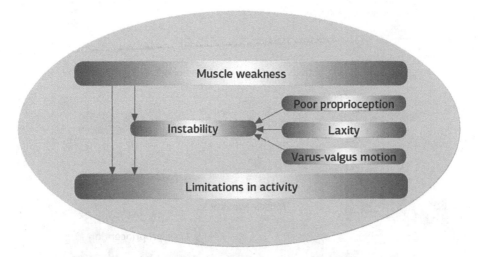

Fig. 1.2 Neuromuscular factors and activity limitations

Integrated Explanatory Model

Muscle weakness is a pivotal factor in both the behavioral explanation and the neuromuscular explanation of activity limitations in OA. These explanatory models can be integrated into a single model with muscle weakness as the common factor. This is illustrated in Fig. 1.3. This integrated model shows that pain and psychological distress induce avoidance of activity; avoidance of activity causes muscle weakness; muscle weakness has a direct impact on activity limitations; and muscle weakness also interacts with poor proprioception, laxity, and varus-valgus motion, causing instability of the knee joint and activity limitations.

Research on these explanations of functional decline in OA has been published as separate papers; the evidence is scattered and an integrative review is missing. The *second objective* of this book is therefore to review recent research on behavioral and neuromuscular factors in functional decline in OA of the knee or hip with a special emphasis on explanatory mechanisms.

Exercise Therapy

Exercise therapy is among the principal interventions in OA of the knee or hip. Systematic reviews have documented that exercise therapy is effective in reducing pain and activity limitations in OA of the knee, and most likely also OA of the hip. All major therapeutic guidelines on OA advise to refer patients for exercise therapy.

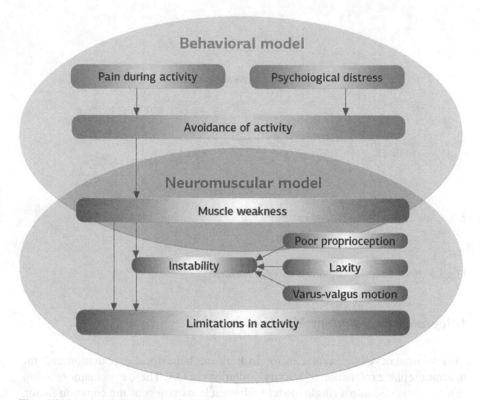

Fig. 1.3 Integrated behavioral and neuromuscular explanation of activity limitations in osteoarthritis

There is a need to further develop exercise therapy. Although clearly effective, the impact of exercise therapy on pain and activity limitations is moderate. Further development of exercise therapy is expected to result in improved outcome. The need for further development of exercise therapy is reinforced by the limitations of other therapeutic interventions in OA. Most pharmacological approaches may suffer from harmful side effects. Surgical interventions are preferably applied in the later stages of the disease, as the survival of orthopedic devices is frequently limited. Against this background, the contribution of exercise therapy and need for further development in this area is obvious.

The previously discussed explanatory models provide important insights for the further development of exercise therapy. The behavioral and neuromuscular models describe specific causes of functional decline in OA. Innovative approaches toward exercise therapy have been developed, targeting these causes of functional decline.

Targeted Exercise Therapy: Physical Activity

The behavioral explanation of activity limitations in OA is based on avoidance of activity; avoidance of activity causes muscle weakness and thereby activity limitations. This suggests that combining exercise therapy with gradually increasing the level of physical activity physical activity will result in less activity limitations. Regular exercise therapy consists of exercises aimed at muscle strengthening, improving range of joint motion, and improving aerobic capacity, and functional exercises aimed at improving activities of daily life such as walking. Combining the gradual increase of physical activity with the more traditional modalities of exercise therapy counteracts the effects of avoidance of activity and will result in a better outcome of exercise therapy.

Targeted Exercise Therapy: Stabilization of the Knee

Improving muscle strength is one of the traditional goals of regular exercise therapy; improved muscle strength results in less activity limitations. The neuro-muscular model of activity limitations in OA suggests that other factors such as poor proprioception and laxity need to be addressed as well. The combination of muscle weakness and poor proprioception or laxity are hypothesized to cause instability of the knee, and thereby activity limitations. This suggests that exercise modalities aimed at improving proprioception and reducing the consequences of laxity need to be incorporated into the more traditional modalities such as muscle strengthening exercise.

Tailored Exercise Therapy: Comorbidity and Overweight

OA is one of the diseases with the highest rate of comorbidity. Comorbidity is defined as any distinct additional clinical entity that has existed or that may occur during the clinical course of a patient who has the index disease (i.e., osteoarthritis) under study [9]. Common comorbidities in OA include coronary diseases, heart failure, hypertension, diabetes, obesity, chronic obstructive pulmonary disease, COPD, chronic pain, depression, and visual and hearing impairments. Comorbidity in OA is associated with more limitations in activities, more pain, and a poor functional prognosis [10, 11].

Comorbidity is associated with the risk of serious adverse events during exercise, e.g., cardiac decompensation. Exercise therapy may need to be adapted in order to avoid these adverse events. In other cases, exercise therapy may need to be adapted in order to optimize efficacy. For example, in the presence of depression or chronic pain, adaptations to exercise therapy are required in order to optimize outcome. Comorbidities may necessitate several adaptations of exercise, which sometimes are even contradictory. The inherent variation and complexity of comorbidities makes clinical reasoning and tailoring of exercise an absolute requirement.

The *third objective* of this book is to review innovative approaches toward exercise therapy, derived from research on behavioral, neuromuscular, and medical factors in functional decline in OA of the knee or hip.

Overview

Part I is a clinical overview of osteoarthritis of the hip or knee. Our knowledge on epidemiology, pathogenesis, and clinical aspects of OA of the knee or hip is summarized in Chap. 2. Chapter 3 summarizes therapeutic options in OA of the knee or hip.

Part II concerns functional decline in OA of the knee or hip. Risk factors for functional decline are summarized in Chap. 4. Two major explanatory models explaining functional decline are reviewed in the next chapters; neuromuscular mechanisms in Chap. 5 and behavioral mechanisms in Chap. 6.

Part III concerns exercise as a therapeutic approach in OA of the knee and hip. Regular exercise therapy is reviewed in Chap. 7, while exercise aiming at neuromuscular mechanisms and behavioral mechanisms is reviewed in Chaps. 8 and 9, respectively. Chapter 10 addresses comorbidity and overweight in OA, and adaptations of exercise therapy required because of comorbidity and overweight.

Chapter 11 concerns concluding remarks.

Terminology

This book relies on the terminology introduced in WHO's International Classification of Functioning (ICF) to describe OA-related disability [12]. The term impairment refers to problems in physiological functions of body systems (e.g., muscle weakness) or anatomical body structures. The term activity limitation refers to difficulties an individual may have in executing tasks or actions (e.g., walking). The term participation restriction refers to problems an individual may experience in involvement in life situations (e.g., a job). The term functioning refers to all body functions, activities, and participation, while disability is similarly an umbrella term for impairments, activity limitations, and participation restrictions. Research on OA-related disability is characterized by a sometimes bewildering lack of standardization of terminology, leading to scientific confusion.

Adoption of the internationally accepted ICF-terminology is essential to facilitate scientific communication, in research on OA-related disability, as well as research in other fields.

References

1. World Health Organization (2008) Global burden of disease. 2004 Update. World Health Organization, Geneva
2. Jordan JM, Helmick CG, Renner JB, Luta G, Dragomir AD, Woodard J et al (2007) Prevalence of knee symptoms and radiographic and symptomatic knee osteoarthritis in African Americans and Caucasians: the Johnston County Osteoarthritis Project. J Rheumatol 34(1):172–180
3. Zhang Y, Jordan JM (2010) Epidemiology of osteoarthritis. Clin Geriatr Med 26(3):355–369
4. Hawker GA, Stewart L, French MR, Cibere J, Jordan JM, March L et al (2008) Understanding the pain experience in hip and knee osteoarthritis–an OARSI/OMERACT initiative. Osteoarthritis Cartilage 16(4):415–422
5. Covinsky KE, Lindquist K, Dunlop DD, Gill TM, Yelin E (2008) Effect of arthritis in middle age on older-age functioning. J Am Geriatr Soc 56(1):23–28
6. van Dijk GM, Dekker J, Veenhof C, van den Ende CH (2006) Course of functional status and pain in osteoarthritis of the hip or knee: a systematic review of the literature. Arthritis Rheum 55(5):779–785
7. Dekker J, van Dijk GM, Veenhof C (2009) Risk factors for functional decline in osteoarthritis of the hip or knee. Curr Opin Rheumatol 21(5):520–524
8. White DK, Keysor JJ, LaValley MP, Lewis CE, Torner JC, Nevitt MC et al (2010) Clinically important improvement in function is common in people with or at high risk of knee OA: the MOST study. J Rheumatol 37(6):1244–1251
9. Feinstein AR (1970) The pre-therapeutic classification of co-morbidity in chronic disease. Chronic Dis 23:455–468
10. van Dijk GM, Veenhof C, Schellevis F, Hulsmans H, Bakker JP, Arwert H et al (2008) Comorbidity, limitations in activities and pain in patients with osteoarthritis of the hip or knee. BMC Musculoskelet Disord 9:95
11. van Dijk GM, Veenhof C, Spreeuwenberg P, Coene N, Burger BJ, van Schaardenburg D et al (2010) Prognosis of limitations in activities in osteoarthritis of the hip or knee: a 3-year cohort study. Arch Phys Med Rehabil 91(1):58–66
12. WHO (2002) Towards a common language for functioning, disability and health: ICF. http://www.who.int/classifications/icf/site/icftemplate cfm

Part I
Osteoarthritis of the Knee or Hip

Chapter 2
Epidemiology, Pathogenesis, and Clinical Aspects of Knee and Hip Osteoarthritis

Diana C. Sanchez-Ramirez, Joost Dekker, and Willem F. Lems

Osteoarthritis (OA) is considered the most common form of arthritis affecting synovial joints [1]. OA is associated with pain and activity limitations [2]. Its overall prevalence is roughly estimated at 151.4 million people worldwide. OA is counted globally as the sixth primary cause of moderate-to-severe disability and the eighth cause of disease burden in the European region [3]. As a consequence, this disease has become not only an important healthcare challenge but also a major public health and socioeconomic concern [4, 5].

Epidemiology

Prevalence. The prevalence of knee (Fig. 2.1) and hip (Fig. 2.2) OA varies according to the criteria used to define the diagnosis and the characteristics of the population studied. For research purposes, OA can be defined pathologically, radiographically, or clinically [6]. The last two classifications are the most commonly used.

Radiological OA refers to the morphological or structural changes within the joint visible on X-rays. Those changes are usually defined using the Kellgren–Lawrence scale (K&L) [8], which is the most widely used radiological classification.

D.C. Sanchez-Ramirez
Faculty of Human Movement Sciences, VU University, Amsterdam, The Netherlands

J. Dekker (✉)
Department of Rehabilitation Medicine, VU University Medical Center, PO Box 7057,
1007 MB Amsterdam, The Netherlands

Department of Psychiatry, VU University Medical Center, Amsterdam, The Netherlands
e-mail: j.dekker@vumc.nl

W.F. Lems
Department of Rheumatology, VU University Medical Center, Amsterdam, The Netherlands

J. Dekker (ed.), *Exercise and Physical Functioning in Osteoarthritis: Medical,*
Neuromuscular and Behavioral Perspectives, Springer Briefs in Specialty Topics in
Behavioral Medicine, DOI 10.1007/978-1-4614-7215-5_2, © The Author(s) 2014

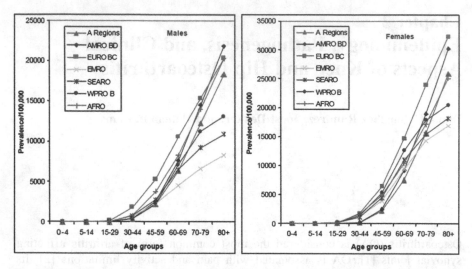

Fig. 2.1 Prevalence of osteoarthritis of the knee, by age, sex, and region, 2000. A Regions = developed countries in North America, Western Europe, Japan, Australia, and New Zealand. AMRO BD = developing countries in the Americas. EURO BC = developing countries in Europe. EMRO = countries in the Eastern Mediterranean and North African regions. SEARO = countries in Southeast Asia. WPRO B = countries in the Western Pacific region. AFRO = countries in sub-Saharan Africa [7]

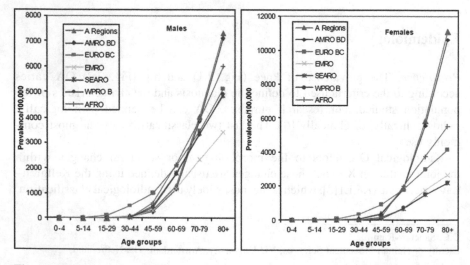

Fig. 2.2 Prevalence of osteoarthritis of the hip, by age, sex, and region, 2000. *Source*: Symmons et al. [7]. Available at: http://www.who.int/healthinfo/statistics/bod_osteoarthritis.pdf

On this scale, the presence and severity of OA is defined according to intra-articular changes such as osteophyte formation (bony projections along joint margins), periarticular ossicles (small bones surrounding the joint surface), thinning of the joint cartilage with narrowing of the intra-articular joint space, and formation of

Table 2.1 Kellgren–Lawrence Grading Scale

Grade 0	No radiographic findings of OA
Grade 1	Doubtful narrowing of joint space and possible osteophytic lipping
Grade 2	Definite osteophytes and possible narrowing of joint space
Grade 3	Moderate multiple osteophytes, definite narrowing of joints space and some sclerosis and possible deformity of bone end
Grade 4	Large osteophytes, marked narrowing of joint space, sever sclerosis deformity of bone end

Source: Kellgren JH, JeffreyMR, Ball J. The epidemiology of chronic rheumatism. Atlas of standard radiographs of arthritis. Oxford, UK: Blackwell Scientific Publications, 1963:vii–11

pseudocystic areas (dilated spaces resembling cysts) with sclerotic (thick) walls. These features are used to define a scale of 5 (0, normal to 4, severe) [9] (Table 2.1; Fig. 2.3). Some disadvantages associated with the K&L classification include the high probability of interobserver variation, low sensibility to changes of the scale and the difficulty to detect the disease in an early stage.

In people older than 80 years, 53 % of women and 33 % of men had radiographic osteoarthritis of the knee, defined as the K&L grade ≥2 [10]. Prevalence of radiographic hip OA was estimated as 27 % among adults aged ≥45 years [8]. Other studies have reported slight variations of these prevalences [8, 11].

Symptomatic OA is considered if in addition to the presence of radiographic changes, the person suffers from joint pain, aching or stiffness [6]. Data from the Johnston county, osteoarthritis project showed prevalence of symptomatic OA of 16.7 % in the knee [12] and 9.2 % in the hip among adults aged ≥45 years [8]. Some variations of symptomatic knee OA prevalence were reported in other American studies [8, 11].

Currently, it is estimated that the prevalence of OA will continue rising worldwide mainly due to the increase in life expectancy and the prevalence of obesity within the population [6, 13].

Incidence. Oliveria et al. [14] calculated the age- and sex-standardized incidence rate for knee OA as 240/100,000 person-years and for hip OA as 88/100,000 person-years. The annual incidence of symptomatic and radiographic knee OA were estimated to increase by 1 % and 2 %, respectively [15].

Progression of Radiographic OA, Symptoms and Activity Limitations. Progression of radiographic OA is generally low, estimated at 4 % per year [15]. Progression is found in the majority of hip and knee OA cases and can be associated with worsening of the symptoms [16]. In osteoarthritic hips, a study documented a slight radiographic progression (K&L grade) compared with high increase on pain scores [17]. On the other hand, after 5 years follow-up, 54 % of individuals with knee pain showed signs of radiographic OA, using knee images and digital analysis of separate quantitative features (i.e., osteophytes and joint space) [18]. These studies demonstrate that the progression of radiological OA and symptoms are not necessarily

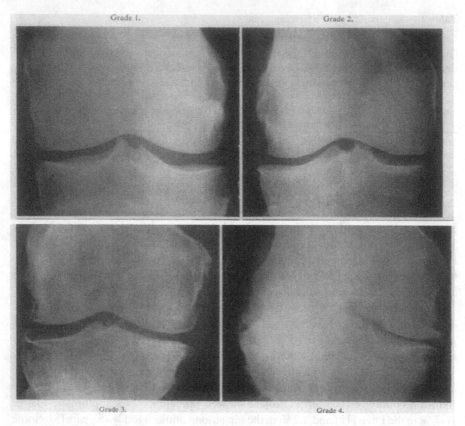

Fig. 2.3 Kellgren–Lawrence Grading Scale. *Source*: Kellgren and Lawrence. Ann. Rheum. Dis. (1957), 16,494

correlated. Interestingly, some authors have reported an improvement in K&L scores and an improvement of symptoms in knee OA patients [19, 20].

Pain and activity limitations in hip or knee OA seem to progress slowly over time, with significant changes being observed after 3 years of follow-up [21]. Holla et al. [22] observed that 48.7 % and 49.7 % of the participants with early knee and hip OA symptoms were classified as experiencing poor outcome on activity limitations after 2 years. Moreover, older age, varus knee alignment, presence of the disease in more than one joint, and presence of radiographic features were detected as predictors of knee OA progression [23].

Knee and hip osteoarthritis have been associated with reduced survival rates [16]. A higher mortality ratio of 1.55 was established in OA patients compared to the general population [24]. Studies have suggested that this phenomenon may result from the combination of several factors such as obesity, a low grade of systemic inflammation, prolonged use of NSAID medicines, and/or lack of physical activity [25].

In general, radiographic and clinical osteoarthritis progress over time [26]. However, there are some cases in which the disease might remain stable or even show some improvements [17, 19, 20]. Unfortunately, the mechanisms underlying disease progression are poorly understood. Therefore, further studies are needed in order to better understand the course of the disease.

Pathogenesis

The pathogenesis of OA has long been mainly related to changes initiated in the articular cartilage. However, recent evidence has suggested the participation of subchondral bone and synovial membrane within the disease's development and progression [10] as illustrated in Fig. 2.4.

The articular cartilage has a unique matrix structure rich in collagen and proteoglycans. This allows cartilage to absorb stress forces, to deform under mechanical load, and to provide a smooth load-bearing surface facilitating the joint's movement [27]. Genetic, biomechanical and biochemical factors may alter the normal functioning of chondrocyte cells promoting a disruption of the equilibrium between the continual formation and breakdown of the cartilaginous matrix, and leading to a failure of the homeostatic balance maintenance [28–30]. As a consequence, the cartilage becomes part of a vicious cycle of depletion resulting in progressive loss of the hyaline cartilage within the joint and usually also

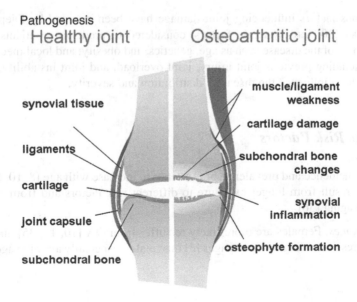

Pathogenesis
Healthy joint   Osteoarthritic joint

synovial tissue

muscle/ligament
weakness

cartilage damage

ligaments

subchondral bone
changes

cartilage

synovial
inflammation

joint capsule

subchondral bone

osteophyte formation

Fig. 2.4 Healthy vs. osteoarthritic joint

leading to underlying subchondral bony changes [28, 30]. Although some evidence supports this disease pathway, this sequence of pathogenesis is still a matter of debate.

Osteochondral changes characteristic of OA disease may occur early during the development of OA and accentuate during the disease progression. Recent evidence suggests subchondral bone as a possible precursor of the cartilage damage rather than being the consequence of it [10, 27]. Moreover, it is suggested that the integrity of the cartilage depends on the mechanical properties of its bony underlying. Therefore, the bone's loss of effective capacity to absorb forces (stiffening of subchondral bone) caused by repetitive microfractures may affect the cartilage's overlay integrity [27]. According to Intema et al. [31], thinning of the subchondral plate is related to cartilage degeneration while trabecular bone changes are related to mechanical loading.

Synovial inflammation may occur as a consequence of posttraumatic joint injury [32] or secondary to the chemical process associated with early or late phases of OA. It usually corresponds to clinical symptoms of joint swelling and pain [10]. Cartilage degeneration might be promoted by the release of catabolic and proinflammatory mediators from the synovial membrane (i.e., IL-1, IL-6, THF-α, etc.) [33] and by the excessive production of the proteolytic enzymes responsible for cartilage breakdown [34]. This vicious cycle might contribute to progressive joint degeneration.

Risk Factors

The various factors influencing joint damage have been grouped by Dieppe and Lohmander [30] into systemic factors, considered to predispose patients to the development of the disease such as age, genetics, and obesity; and local mechanical factors including previous joint injury, joint overload, and joint instability, which are thought to influence the disease's distribution and severity.

Systemic Risk Factors

Age. The incidence and prevalence of OA tends to increase with age [8, 10, 11, 35]. This may result from longer exposure to different risk factors and from changes related to aging [36].

Sex Hormones. Females are more likely to suffer from OA [10, 11, 35] and show more aggressive radiographic changes [5] than males, especially after the age of 50.

It is suggested that this phenomenon is related to hormonal changes occurring after the menopause [27].

Genetic Predisposition. Higher risk of OA has been related to a genetic predisposition [33] through chromosomal loci and gene variations associations [30]. However, identification of osteoarthritis susceptibility loci has not been as successful as expected [37], and further research related to this risk factor is needed.

Race and Ethnicity. Differences in OA prevalence linked to race and ethnicity have been identified [6, 38, 39]. Anatomical racial/ethnic characteristics may explain some of the variations [6].

Vitamin D. There is evidence suggesting that vitamin D may influence the course of OA by causing some effects on bone and cartilage [40]. However, recent studies have found vitamin D to be more likely to be associated to the level of pain but not to radiographic changes in knee OA [41].

Excess Weight and Obesity. This factor is strongly related to OA [6, 35, 42, 43]. The mechanism influencing the relationship is not clear. However, studies have suggested that this correlation is not only the result of mechanical overload, particularly at the hips and knees, but also the result of the influence of some systemic factors [44, 45] such as the production of the so-called adipocytokines in abdominal fat mass. This concept is supported by the presence of OA in nonweight-bearing joints such as hand joints in obese individuals.

Local Mechanical Risk Factors

Previous Injury. Previous joint injuries, such as transarticular fractures, meniscal tear, or anterior ligament injury, are important risk factors linked to the development of knee OA [6, 46, 47]. This is usually referenced as posttraumatic osteoarthritis and represents approximately 12 % of all OA in the hip and knee [48].

Physical Activity. Regular practice or intense sporting activities may be considered a risk factor for development of OA [47]. However, the evidence on engagement in regular physical activity and the risk for the development of OA is conflicting [6]. Also, some occupational activities requiring heavy lifting or constant kneeling have been correlated to OA of the hip and knee, respectively [49].

Muscle Weakness and Malalignment. Formerly, these factors were considered a consequence rather than a cause of OA [30]. However, recently quadriceps weakness has been considered as a potential risk factor for symptomatic knee OA [50]. Similarly, knee malalignment has been related to a higher risk of development and progression of knee OA due to intra-articular alterations of load distribution [6].

Diagnosis and Diagnostic Criteria

Clinical Symptoms and Signs

Joint pain is the main reason for the initial visit to the general practitioner [6]. Pain is described as a continuous dull or aching pain, which is interspersed with unpredictable short episodes of high intensity [51]. Typically, this pain increases during weight-bearing activities and is relieved with rest. In later stages, pain occurs at gradually shorter walking distances and may finally even occur in rest and at night. Pain in OA is sometimes accompanied by joint swelling or hydrops, a mild inflammatory phase easier to diagnose in knee than in hip OA. Stiffness is another OA symptom present in the morning, in the evening, or after periods of inactivity, which lasts for a short period of time (less than 30 min) [30, 51]. Additional signs related to OA include bony enlargement, impaired range of joint motion, crepitus on motion, tenderness on pressure, pain on motion, joint effusion, malalignment, and/or joint deformity [6, 27]. Moreover, osteoarthritis patients experience activity limitations that affect their ability to live independently.

Painful osteoarthritis is usually difficult to differentiate from other causes of joint pain such as referred pain, other periarticular pathologies, and somatization [30]. However, the use of a complete patient history analysis and physical examination is usually enough to make an accurate diagnosis. Sometimes laboratory test and X-rays are performed to assist the physician in establishing a precise diagnosis or to reassure the patient.

Anamnesis. Usually healthcare providers' ask for a description of the clinical symptoms described above such as joint pain and stiffness. Also, information related to heredity, past joint trauma, and occupational risks might help to direct the diagnosis.

Physical Examination. Physical examination is complementary to the anamnesis. It should be guided by the ACR criteria (see diagnostic criteria below). This exam is intended for the detection of additional signs including bony enlargement, impaired range of joint motion, tenderness, pain on motion, joint effusion, muscle strength, malalignment, and joint deformity [28].

Imaging. Radiographic images are relatively cheap, fast, and easy to take. That is why they are largely used for diagnosis and follow-up of the disease progression. However, X-rays show only a limited two-dimensional view of the joint and some relevant features might be missed [10, 28]. Magnetic resonance imaging (MRI) is a more complete type of imaging, which offers a three-dimensional overview of the different structures in the joint. However, it is a time-consuming and more expensive diagnostic test [10]. Furthermore, the large amount of data generated by MRI may be difficult to report and to interpret. Computerized tomography also offers a three-dimensional view of the joint, but the radiation exposure and the high cost involved prevent its common use [10].

Table 2.2 American College of Rheumatology radiological and clinical criteria for osteoarthritis of the knee and hip

Hip (clinical and radiographic)
Osteoarthritis if 1, 2, 3 or 1, 2, 4 or 1, 3, 4 are present:
1   Hip pain for most days of previous month
2   Erythrocyte sedimentation rate of less than 20 mm in the first hour
3   Femoral or acetabular osteophytes on radiographs
4   Hip joint space narrowing on radiographs
Knee (clinical)
Osteoarthritis if 1, 2, 3, 4 or 1, 2, 5 or 1, 4, 5 are present:
1   Knee pain for most days of previous month
2   Crepitus on active joint motion
3   Morning stiffness lasting 30 min or less
4   Age 38 years or older
5   Bony enlargement of the knee on examination
Knee (clinical and radiographic)
Osteoarthritis if 1, 2 or 1, 3, 5, 6 or 1, 4, 5, 6 are present:
1   Knee pain for most days of previous month
2   Osteophytes at joint margins on radiographs
3   Synovial fluid typical of osteoarthritis (laboratory)
4   Age 40 years or older
5   Crepitus on active joint motion
6   Morning stiffness lasting 30 min or less

Bijlsma JW, Berenbaum F, Lafeber FP. Osteoarthritis: an update with relevance for clinical practice. Lancet 2011 Jun 18; 377(9783):2115–26

Laboratory Tests. Most routine blood tests are normal in patients with uncomplicated osteoarthritis, and thus it is not absolutely necessary to perform these tests. To assist the physician and to reassure the patient, conventional blood test analysis, like erythrocyte sedimentation rate (ESR), might be used to differentiate OA from other inflammatory rheumatic diseases (i.e., rheumatoid arthritis or gout) [10].

Diagnostic Criteria. The American College of Rheumatology (ACR) has published classification guidelines presenting the diagnostic criteria for idiopathic knee OA in 1986 [52] and hip OA in 1991 [53, 54]. The clinical criteria for OA of knee and hip formulated by the ACR are summarized in Table 2.2.

Phenotypes

Currently, etiology and progression of OA are not fully understood. Therefore, the identification of patients most likely to develop the disease or those at risk of rapid disease progression is highly relevant. Consequently, the characterization of the OA patients according to common phenotypes is considered of clinical importance.

In an attempt to better direct the disease treatment, some authors have proposed a categorization intended to group the heterogeneous patients' features following their most relevant characteristics. In knee OA patients, five phenotypes were identified by Knoop et al. [55] based on clinically relevant patient characteristics: "minimal joint disease phenotype," "strong muscle phenotype," "nonobese and weak muscle phenotype," "obese and weak muscle phenotype," and "depressive phenotype." Bijlsma et al. [10] proposed differentiating the clinical phenotypes of OA according to posttraumatic, metabolic, ageing, genetic, or pain. At this time, the definition of the most appropriate disease phenotypes is still an ongoing debate. There is considerable interest in this topic, because of the need to understand disease progression.

Conclusion

OA is a chronic disease with a high and increasing prevalence and incidence. Because of the moderate effects of nonpharmacological and pharmacological treatments [56], the prevention through the counteraction of risk factors and the detection of early signs should be highly prioritized. However, the discrepancy between symptoms and radiological features in addition to the absence of clear parameters to guide early identification of OA usually ends up in establishing the diagnosis of OA at a late stage, when there are already several tissue abnormalities. Further studies are needed in order to better understand the disease's etiology and progression, especially focusing on early OA.

References

1. Pendleton A, Arden N, Dougados M, Doherty M, Bannwarth B, Bijlsma JW et al (2000) EULAR recommendations for the management of knee osteoarthritis: report of a task force of the Standing Committee for International Clinical Studies Including Therapeutic Trials (ESCISIT). Ann Rheum Dis 59(12):936–944
2. Conaghan PG, Dickson J, Grant RL (2008) Care and management of osteoarthritis in adults: summary of NICE guidance. BMJ 336(7642):502–503
3. World Health Organization (2008) Global burden of disease. 2004 Update. World Health Organization, Geneva
4. Bitton R (2009) The economic burden of osteoarthritis. Am J Manag Care 15(8 Suppl): S230–S235
5. Srikanth VK, Fryer JL, Zhai G, Winzenberg TM, Hosmer D, Jones G (2005) A meta-analysis of sex differences prevalence, incidence and severity of osteoarthritis. Osteoarthritis Cartilage 13(9):769–781
6. Zhang Y, Jordan JM (2010) Epidemiology of osteoarthritis. Clin Geriatr Med 26(3):355–369
7. Symmons D, Mathers C, Pfleger B (2003) Global burden of osteoarthritis in the year 2000. World Health Organization, Geneva

8. Lawrence RC, Felson DT, Helmick CG, Arnold LM, Choi H, Deyo RA et al (2008) Estimates of the prevalence of arthritis and other rheumatic conditions in the United States. Part II. Arthritis Rheum 58(1):26–35
9. Kellgren JH, Lawrence JS (1957) Radiological assessment of osteo-arthrosis. Ann Rheum Dis 16:494–502
10. Bijlsma JW, Berenbaum F, Lafeber FP (2011) Osteoarthritis: an update with relevance for clinical practice. Lancet 377(9783):2115–2126
11. Dillon CF, Rasch EK, Gu Q, Hirsch R (2006) Prevalence of knee osteoarthritis in the United States: arthritis data from the Third National Health and Nutrition Examination Survey 1991–94. J Rheumatol 33(11):2271–2279
12. Jordan JM, Helmick CG, Renner JB, Luta G, Dragomir AD, Woodard J et al (2007) Prevalence of knee symptoms and radiographic and symptomatic knee osteoarthritis in African Americans and Caucasians: the Johnston County Osteoarthritis Project. J Rheumatol 34(1):172–180
13. Duncan R, Peat G, Thomas E, Hay EM, Croft P (2011) Incidence, progression and sequence of development of radiographic knee osteoarthritis in a symptomatic population. Ann Rheum Dis 70(11):1944–1948
14. Oliveria SA, Felson DT, Reed JI, Cirillo PA, Walker AM (1995) Incidence of symptomatic hand, hip, and knee osteoarthritis among patients in a health maintenance organization. Arthritis Rheum 38(8):1134–1141
15. Felson DT, Zhang Y, Hannan MT, Naimark A, Weissman BN, Aliabadi P et al (1995) The incidence and natural history of knee osteoarthritis in the elderly. The Framingham Osteoarthritis Study. Arthritis Rheum 38(10):1500–1505
16. Hochberg MC (1996) Prognosis of osteoarthritis. Ann Rheum Dis 55(9):685–688
17. Ledingham J, Dawson S, Preston B, Milligan G, Doherty M (1993) Radiographic progression of hospital referred osteoarthritis of the hip. Ann Rheum Dis 52(4):263–267
18. Kinds MB, Marijnissen AC, Vincken KL, Viergever MA, Drossaers-Bakker KW, Bijlsma JW et al (2012) Evaluation of separate quantitative radiographic features adds to the prediction of incident radiographic osteoarthritis in individuals with recent onset of knee pain: 5-year follow-up in the CHECK cohort. Osteoarthritis Cartilage 20(6):548–556
19. Ledingham J, Regan M, Jones A, Doherty M (1995) Factors affecting radiographic progression of knee osteoarthritis. Ann Rheum Dis 54(1):53–58
20. Spector TD, Dacre JE, Harris PA, Huskisson EC (1992) Radiological progression of osteoarthritis: an 11 year follow up study of the knee. Ann Rheum Dis 51(10):1107–1110
21. van Dijk GM, Dekker J, Veenhof C, Van den Ende CH (2006) Course of functional status and pain in osteoarthritis of the hip or knee: a systematic review of the literature. Arthritis Rheum 55(5):779–785
22. Holla JF, Steultjens MP, Roorda LD, Heymans MW, Ten WS, Dekker J (2010) Prognostic factors for the two-year course of activity limitations in early osteoarthritis of the hip and/or knee. Arthritis Care Res (Hoboken) 62(10):1415–1425
23. Chapple CM, Nicholson H, Baxter GD, Abbott JH (2011) Patient characteristics that predict progression of knee osteoarthritis: a systematic review of prognostic studies. Arthritis Care Res (Hoboken) 63(8):1115–1125
24. Nuesch E, Dieppe P, Reichenbach S, Williams S, Iff S, Juni P (2011) All cause and disease specific mortality in patients with knee or hip osteoarthritis: population based cohort study. BMJ 342:d1165
25. Cooper C, Arden NK (2011) Excess mortality in osteoarthritis. BMJ 342:d1407
26. Jordan KM, Arden NK, Doherty M, Bannwarth B, Bijlsma JW, Dieppe P et al (2003) EULAR Recommendations 2003: an evidence based approach to the management of knee osteoarthritis: Report of a Task Force of the Standing Committee for International Clinical Studies Including Therapeutic Trials (ESCISIT). Ann Rheum Dis 62(12):1145–1155
27. Creamer P, Hochberg MC (1997) Osteoarthritis. Lancet 350(9076):503–508
28. Michael JW, Schluter-Brust KU, Eysel P (2010) The epidemiology, etiology, diagnosis, and treatment of osteoarthritis of the knee. Dtsch Arztebl Int 107(9):152–162

29. Goldring MB (2000) The role of the chondrocyte in osteoarthritis. Arthritis Rheum 43(9):1916–1926
30. Dieppe PA, Lohmander LS (2005) Pathogenesis and management of pain in osteoarthritis. Lancet 365(9463):965–973
31. Intema F, Hazewinkel HA, Gouwens D, Bijlsma JW, Weinans H, Lafeber FP et al (2010) In early OA, thinning of the subchondral plate is directly related to cartilage damage: results from a canine ACLT-meniscectomy model. Osteoarthritis Cartilage 18(5):691–698
32. Goldring MB, Otero M (2011) Inflammation in osteoarthritis. Curr Opin Rheumatol 23(5):471–478
33. Madry H, Luyten FP, Facchini A (2012) Biological aspects of early osteoarthritis. Knee Surg Sports Traumatol Arthrosc 20(3):407–422
34. Sellam J, Berenbaum F (2010) The role of synovitis in pathophysiology and clinical symptoms of osteoarthritis. Nat Rev Rheumatol 6(11):625–635
35. Fransen M, Bridgett L, March L, Hoy D, Penserga E, Brooks P (2011) The epidemiology of osteoarthritis in Asia. Int J Rheum Dis 14(2):113–121
36. Loeser RF (2011) Aging and osteoarthritis. Curr Opin Rheumatol 23(5):492–496
37. Loughlin J (2011) Genetics of osteoarthritis. Curr Opin Rheumatol 23(5):479–483
38. Zhang Y, Xu L, Nevitt MC, Aliabadi P, Yu W, Qin M et al (2001) Comparison of the prevalence of knee osteoarthritis between the elderly Chinese population in Beijing and whites in the United States: the Beijing Osteoarthritis Study. Arthritis Rheum 44(9):2065–2071
39. Nelson AE, Braga L, Renner JB, Atashili J, Woodard J, Hochberg MC et al (2010) Characterization of individual radiographic features of hip osteoarthritis in African American and White women and men: the Johnston County Osteoarthritis Project. Arthritis Care Res (Hoboken) 62(2):190–197
40. Felson DT, Niu J, Clancy M, Aliabadi P, Sack B, Guermazi A et al (2007) Low levels of vitamin D and worsening of knee osteoarthritis: results of two longitudinal studies. Arthritis Rheum 56(1):129–136
41. Muraki S, Dennison E, Jameson K, Boucher BJ, Akune T, Yoshimura N et al (2011) Association of vitamin D status with knee pain and radiographic knee osteoarthritis. Osteoarthritis Cartilage 19(11):1301–1306
42. Jiang L, Tian W, Wang Y, Rong J, Bao C, Liu Y et al (2012) Body mass index and susceptibility to knee osteoarthritis: a systematic review and meta-analysis. Joint Bone Spine 79(3):291–297
43. Sowers M (2001) Epidemiology of risk factors for osteoarthritis: systemic factors. Curr Opin Rheumatol 13(5):447–451
44. Conde J, Scotece M, Gomez R, Lopez V, Gomez-Reino JJ, Gualillo O (2011) Adipokines and osteoarthritis: novel molecules involved in the pathogenesis and progression of disease. Arthritis 2011:203901
45. Rai MF, Sandell L (2011) Inflammatory mediators: tracing links between obesity and osteoarthritis. Crit Rev Eukaryot Gene Expr 21(2):131–142
46. Moretz JA III, Harlan SD, Goodrich J, Walters R (1984) Long-term followup of knee injuries in high school football players. Am J Sports Med 12(4):298–300
47. Kujala UM, Kettunen J, Paananen H, Aalto T, Battie MC, Impivaara O et al (1995) Knee osteoarthritis in former runners, soccer players, weight lifters, and shooters. Arthritis Rheum 38(4):539–546
48. Kramer WC, Hendricks KJ, Wang J (2011) Pathogenetic mechanisms of posttraumatic osteoarthritis: opportunities for early intervention. Int J Clin Exp Med 4(4):285–298
49. Rossignol M, Leclerc A, Allaert FA, Rozenberg S, Valat JP, Avouac B et al (2005) Primary osteoarthritis of hip, knee, and hand in relation to occupational exposure. Occup Environ Med 62(11):772–777
50. Slemenda C, Brandt KD, Heilman DK, Mazzuca S, Braunstein EM, Katz BP et al (1997) Quadriceps weakness and osteoarthritis of the knee. Ann Intern Med 127(2):97–104

51. Hawker GA, Stewart L, French MR, Cibere J, Jordan JM, March L et al (2008) Understanding the pain experience in hip and knee osteoarthritis–an OARSI/OMERACT initiative. Osteoarthritis Cartilage 16(4):415–422
52. Altman R, Asch E, Bloch D, Bole G, Borenstein D, Brandt K et al (1986) Development of criteria for the classification and reporting of osteoarthritis. Classification of osteoarthritis of the knee. Diagnostic and Therapeutic Criteria Committee of the American Rheumatism Association. Arthritis Rheum 29(8):1039–1049
53. Altman R, Alarcon G, Appelrouth D, Bloch D, Borenstein D, Brandt K et al (1991) The American College of Rheumatology criteria for the classification and reporting of osteoarthritis of the hip. Arthritis Rheum 34(5):505–514
54. Peat G, Thomas E, Duncan R, Wood L, Hay E, Croft P (2006) Clinical classification criteria for knee osteoarthritis: performance in the general population and primary care. Ann Rheum Dis 65(10):1363–1367
55. Knoop J, van der Leeden LM, Thorstensson CA, Roorda LD, Lems WF, Knol DL et al (2011) Identification of phenotypes with different clinical outcomes in knee osteoarthritis: data from the osteoarthritis initiative. Arthritis Care Res (Hoboken) 63(11):1535–1542
56. Hochberg MC, Altman RD, April KT, Benkhalti M, Guyatt G, McGowan J et al (2012) American College of Rheumatology 2012 recommendations for the use of nonpharmacologic and pharmacologic therapies in osteoarthritis of the hand, hip, and knee. Arthritis Care Res (Hoboken) 64(4):455–474

Chapter 3
Therapeutic Options in Osteoarthritis of the Hip or Knee

Martijn Gerritsen, Ramon E. Voorneman, Joost Dekker, and Willem F. Lems

Osteoarthritis (OA) of the hip or knee is a frequent cause of joint pain and disability, especially in the elderly [1]. It leads to limitations in activities of daily life and eventually to restrictions in social and occupational participation. Treatment should be aimed at reduction of pain and stiffness, minimizing disability, and improvement of quality of life, and prevention or inhibition of disease progression. Unfortunately, at present, there are no disease-modifying treatments for OA that can slow the progression of joint damage. In general, therapy in osteoarthritis of the hip or knee consists of nonpharmacological, pharmacological, and/or surgical interventions. A combination of pharmacological and nonpharmacological treatments is universally recommended in current guidelines for the management of hip and knee OA [2, 3]. In the following chapter these interventions will be discussed.

Nonpharmacological Therapy

Nonpharmacological interventions in patients with OA of hip and knee are of great importance, since drugs that slow disease progression are not available. Furthermore, pharmacological therapy frequently leads to side effects, especially in the presence of comorbid conditions, and surgical interventions are being reserved for end-stage OA.

M. Gerritsen • R.E. Voorneman
Department of Rheumatology | Reade, Amsterdam, The Netherlands

J. Dekker (✉)
Department of Rehabilitation Medicine, VU University Medical Center, PO Box 7057, 1007 MB Amsterdam, The Netherlands

Department of Psychiatry, VU University Medical Center, Amsterdam, The Netherlands
e-mail: j.dekker@vumc.nl

W.F. Lems
Department of Rheumatology, VU University Medical Center, Amsterdam, The Netherlands

J. Dekker (ed.), *Exercise and Physical Functioning in Osteoarthritis: Medical, Neuromuscular and Behavioral Perspectives*, Springer Briefs in Specialty Topics in Behavioral Medicine, DOI 10.1007/978-1-4614-7215-5_3, © The Author(s) 2014

Provision of information and education about OA, the objectives of treatment, and the importance of changes in lifestyle, regular exercise, pacing of activities, weight reduction, and other measures to unload damaged joints, are considered obligatory for all patients. However, the effect-size of these interventions is small on the reduction of pain [2, 3] and no improvement was found on activity limitations [4]. The emphasis of education should be on self-management [2].

Obesity is strongly associated with the development of OA. This association is evident in knee OA [5] but less clear in OA of the hip [6]. Weight loss in obese patients with knee OA has a positive effect on pain and stiffness with small effect sizes and a positive effect on functional improvement with a moderate effect size [2, 7–10]. The combination of a diet and exercise was shown to be the most effective intervention [9]. To date, no randomized controlled trials have been published to confirm similar beneficial effects of weight reduction in patients with OA of the hip. It seems warranted, however to expect a positive effect of weight loss on symptoms in these patients. Therefore, patients with knee or hip OA that are overweight should be encouraged to lose weight and maintain their weight at a lower level [2, 4].

The effects of exercise therapy are discussed in greater detail in Part III. In brief, exercise is a core recommendation in patients with knee OA. Exercise aimed at quadriceps muscle strengthening, improving aerobic endurance, and joint mobility has a small to moderate positive effect on pain and activity limitations [11, 12]. In OA of the hip, there is less extensive evidence of a positive effect of exercise therapy [13]. Still, it is generally accepted that exercise is also beneficial for patients with hip OA. The above-mentioned effects are mainly short-term effects. To conserve long-term effectiveness, it seems important to offer follow-up sessions [14]. To increase the effect of exercise therapy, additional targeted therapies are being developed, aimed at correction of factors underlying functional decline in OA, such as instability, avoidance of activity, and depressed mood. Exercise aimed at neuro-muscular and behavioral mechanisms is extensively described in Part II.

Osteoarthritis of the knee can result in varus or valgus deformation, which opens up the possibility to perform an osteotomy. Deformation has been shown to be a risk factor for disease progression and loss of function [15]. A knee brace can reduce pain, improve stability and the performance of activities, and reduce the risk of falling [16, 17]. Indeed, an increased risk of falling in OA patients has been documented versus healthy controls [18]. Insoles can be of benefit in patients with hip or knee OA because of the reduction of pain and activity limitations. There is, however, not enough evidence from controlled studies to advocate the use of insoles [2, 4]. On the other hand, every patient with hip or knee OA should receive advice concerning appropriate footwear. Walking aids, like a cane or crutch in the contralateral hand, can reduce pain in OA of the hip or knee. Evidence on the positive effect of a cane on pain, activity limitations, and quality of life has been recently obtained [19].

The effect of electromagnetic therapy in knee OA has not been studied extensively. Improvement in activity limitations was modest and there was no significant efficacy for reduction of pain [20]. Thermotherapy is recommended in some guidelines, although there was no significant effect on pain or on activity limitations [2]. Transcutaneous electrical nerve stimulation (TENS) has short-term efficacy in providing clinically significant pain relief in patients with knee OA and no serious adverse effects were reported [21]. In a meta-analysis, acupuncture was shown to be superior to controls with a moderate relief of pain and improvement in the performance of activities. The effect was lower in blinded trials and also diminished with time [22].

Pharmacological Therapy

Acetaminophen, in doses up to 3–4 g/day is recommended for the initial treatment of mild-to-moderate pain in patients with knee or hip OA because of its safety and efficacy. It was shown to be superior to placebo in reducing pain, although the effect size is small. Acetaminophen has no significant effect on stiffness or functioning in patients with symptomatic knee OA. Acetaminophen in recommended dosages is safe. However, upon chronic use in high dosages (>3 g/day), it may have upper gastrointestinal side effects, lead to mild impairment in renal function, and hypertension [2, 3]. It is also important to realize that it may lead to fatal liver damage when toxic dosages are used, for instance in tentamen suicidi.

In case of insufficient pain relief on acetaminophen, a nonsteroidal anti-inflammatory drug (NSAID) can be added or used as a substitute. NSAIDs are inhibitors of the enzyme cyclooxygenase (COX) of which two isoforms exist; COX-1 and COX-2. In general, NSAIDs can be divided in nonselective agents that inhibit both isoforms and COX-2 selective agents, the so-called coxibs.

NSAIDs were shown to be superior to acetaminophen for pain relief in patients with lower limb joint OA. Effect-sizes in general, however, were small [23]. There is no difference in efficacy between various agents. Efficacy is dose dependent [4].

NSAIDs are associated with significantly more side effects than acetaminophen [24]. These agents can cause, for example, serious gastrointestinal (GI) side effects like peptic ulcers, perforations, and bleeds. In patients with increased GI risk, either a COX-2 selective agent or a nonselective NSAID with coprescription of a proton-pump inhibitor or misoprostol for gastroprotection should be considered [25]. Another concern of NSAIDs is the increased cardiovascular (CV) risk. The overall CV risk associated with coxibs was not significantly greater than that associated with conventional nonselective NSAIDs [26]. In patients with a history of myocardial infarction or a cerebrovascular event, it is unsafe and thus contraindicated to prescribe NSAIDs or coxibs for any period of time. Naproxen seems to be the only exception to this [27]. The current advice from the European Agency for the Evaluation of Medicinal Products (EMEA) is that coxibs are contraindicated in patients with ischemic heart disease or stroke and that caution is needed when prescribing these agents to patients with traditional risk factors for heart disease [28]. In general, to minimize the risk of side effects, NSAIDs should be used at the lowest effective dose and for the shortest duration.

In some countries, topical NSAIDs are frequently used by patients with OA. There is a small and short-term effect of these agents on pain [29]. Overall, topical NSAIDs are safe and do not show more side effects than acetaminophen.

Opioid analgesics can be considered in patients with persistent pain despite treatment with NSAIDs or coxibs with or without acetaminophen. In addition, they can be used in patients at high risk of side effects from NSAIDs or coxibs. Finally, inoperable patients can benefit from opioids. Opioid analgesics showed moderate efficacy in pain reduction and in improving the performance of activities, with acceptable safety in short-term trials [30]. The beneficial effects of opioids, however, are often limited by frequent gastrointestinal side effects such as nausea and constipation [31]. There have been no long-term trials of the use of opioids in patients with OA or comparative studies between NSAIDs and opioids.

Glucosamine sulfate and chondroitin sulfate are both constituents of the matrix of healthy cartilage and used as supplements by patients with OA. Their use has been subject of great controversy. To summarize the available evidence, glucosamine sulfate was not more effective than placebo for pain relief or functional improvement [32, 33], except perhaps for the trial with glucosamine from Rotta Pharm [34]. On the other hand, little risk is associated with their use. Therefore, if a patient wants to use glucosamine sulfate, a sufficient dose of 1,500 mg once daily should be prescribed. If no response is apparent within 3 months treatment should be discontinued.

There is no evidence for significant relief of pain with chondroitin sulfate [3]. On the other hand, this supplement may have structure-modifying effects. A small but significant reduction in the rate of decline of joint space narrowing per year was demonstrated in patients treated with chondroitin sulfate compared with placebo [35, 36].

Structure-modifying effects of alendronate, risedronate, and strontium ranelate have been investigated. Although risedronate reduced markers of cartilage degradation and bone resorption, it did not have a substantial effect on radiological progression of knee OA [37]. Alendronate and strontium ranelate were associated with less spinal osteoarthritis progression compared to placebo in post hoc analysis of pivotal trials [38, 39], not indicating that these drugs should be prescribed for the prevention of progressive osteoarthritis, but that more research is warranted. Recently, it was shown in a randomised, placebo-controlled trial in patients with knee osteoarthritis, that the use of strontiumranelate was associated with a lower radiological jont space narrowing, and with a lower WOMAC(pain) score. Although the effect seems to be relatively small, these data are strongly emphasizing that bone-active drugs might have an effect in osteoarthritis [40].

Intra-articular injections with corticosteroids can be used in the treatment of hip and especially knee OA and should be considered when patients have persistent pain despite anti-inflammatory agents and in case of knee OA, when patients have effusion or other physical signs of local inflammation [2]. The effect size for pain relief was moderate, although short lived and the performance of activities was not significantly improved. Repeated injections prolonged the response up to 1 year [41].

Hyaluronic acid is a large molecular-weight glycosaminoglycan that is a constituent of normal synovial cartilage. Injection of intra-articular hyaluronate has been suggested to be of benefit in patients with knee or hip OA. The effect is characterized by delayed onset but prolonged duration. Injections with hyaluronic acid showed asymptomatic benefit when compared to intra-articular injections of corticosteroids [3]. In a recent randomized placebo-controlled trial, repeated cycles of intra-articular hyaluronic acid injections were confirmed to improve knee osteo-arthritis symptoms and even a marked carry-over effect was noticed [42].

Inhibition of nerve growth factor (NGF) through the monoclonal antibody tanezumab was shown to significantly reduce pain in OA of the knee compared to placebo [43]. It appeared as a very promising approach, but the trials with this agent have been discontinued for the moment because of progressively worsening of OA and even bone necrosis requiring total joint arthroplasty. These side effects are thought to be related to injury from excessive loading of the joint due to the absence of pain [44]. However, new trials with monoclonal antibodies against NGF are under way.

Surgery

Surgical options for OA include total joint replacement, unicompartmental knee replacement, and alternative approaches like arthroscopic lavage and debridement, nettoyage with subchondral drilling or microfracture, and osteotomy [4]. In general, surgery should be reserved for patients with insufficient pain relief and functional improvement to maximal conservative treatment.

Total hip and total knee arthroplasty are appropriate surgical procedures to reduce pain and restore the performance of activities [45]. In addition, total joint replacement was shown to be more cost-effective than the current pharmacological treatments [46]. The need for revision, on the other hand, after 10–15 years is an issue, especially in younger OA patients. Cumulative revision rates at 10 years following total hip arthroplasty and total knee arthroplasty for OA were 7 % [47] and 10 % [48], respectively. Other drawbacks are perioperative complications and persisting complaints in up to 15 % of patients [49]. Total joint replacement should therefore be delayed as long as possible, especially in younger patients. Despite these drawbacks and considerations, the number of total hip and knee replacements increased significantly in the Netherlands [50], indicating the increasing prevalence of OA and insufficient effectiveness of conservative treatment. It also stresses the need for innovative, targeted conservative treatment strategies.

Approximately, one-third of patients with knee OA have a disease that is largely restricted to a single compartment. In these patients, knee pain and the performance of activities were comparable 5 years after unicompartimental knee replacement and total knee arthroplasty, but the range of motion was better after the first procedure. Complication rates and survival were similar [51].

Osteotomy should be considered in young adults with symptomatic hip OA, especially in the presence of dysplasia [52]. For the young and physically active patient with significant symptoms from unicompartmental knee OA, high tibial osteotomy may offer an alternative intervention that delays the need for joint replacement some 10 years [53].

In a randomized controlled trial, no positive effects of arthroscopic lavage and debridement were demonstrated in knee OA on pain or quality of life up to 2 years after surgery [54]. There are no studies investigating this technique in OA of the hip. Nettoyage with subchondral drilling or microfracture might result in pain reduction, although effect size and duration are unclear [4].

Conclusion

Therapeutic options in OA of the hip or knee are predominantly symptomatic, since treatment strategies that prevent radiological progression are not yet available. Nowadays, the effects of exercise therapy are limited, but there are hardly any side effects. To increase the effect of exercise therapy, additional targeted therapies are being developed, aimed at correction of factors underlying functional decline in OA such as instability, avoidance of activity, and depressed mood. Acetaminophen is the first choice in pharmacological therapy, because of its favorable safety profile. NSAIDs and coxibs are more effective but are associated with potentially severe GI or cardiovascular side effects. The effect of opioids has not been investigated intensively, but these agents can be used in case of refractory pain. New therapeutic options include the use of bone sparing drugs and that of antibodies against nerve growth factor; further investigations in these directions seem to be worthwhile.

References

1. Sharma L et al (2006) Epidemiology of osteoarthritis: an update. Curr Opin Rheumatol 18:147–156
2. Zhang W et al (2008) OARSI recommendations for the management of hip and knee osteoarthritis, part II: OARSI evidence-based, expert consensus guidelines. Osteoarthritis Cartilage 16:137–162
3. Zhang W et al (2010) OARSI recommendations for the management of hip and knee osteoarthritis, part III: changes in evidence following systematic cumulative update of research published through January 2009 Osteoarthritis Cartilage 18:476–499
4. Nederlandse Orthopedische Vereniging (2007) Richtlijn Diagnostiek en behandeling van heup en Knie Artrose. CBO, Utrecht
5. Felson DT et al (1988) Obesity and knee osteoarthritis: the Framingham study. Ann Intern Med 109:18–24
6. Lievense AM et al (2002) Influence of obesity on the development of osteoarthritis of the hip: a systematic review. Rheumatology 41:1155–1162
7. Christensen R et al (2005) Weight loss: the treatment of choice for knee osteoarthritis? A randomized trial. Osteoarthritis Cartilage 13:20–27
8. Messier SP et al (2004) Exercise and dietary weight loss in overweight and obese older adults with knee osteoarthritis: the arthritis, diet, and activity promotion trial. Arthritis Rheum 50:1501–1510

9. Richette PJ et al (2011) Beneficial effects of massive weight loss on symptoms, joint biomarkers and systemic inflammation in obese patients with knee OA. Ann Rheum Dis 70:139–144

10. Christensen R et al (2007) Effect of weight reduction in obese patients diagnosed with knee osteoarthritis: a systematic review and meta-analysis. Ann Rheum Dis 66:433–439

11. Fransen M, Mc Connell S (2008) Exercise for osteoarthritis of the knee. Cochrane Database Syst Rev 4:CD004376

12. Jamvedt G et al (2008) Physical therapy interventions for patients with osteoarthritis of the knee: an overview of systematic reviews. Phys Ther 88:123–136

13. Fransen M et al (2010) Does land-based exercise reduce pain and disability associated with hip osteoarthritis ? A meta-analysis of randomized controlled trials. Osteoarthritis Cartilage 18:613–620

14. Pisters MF et al (2007) Long-term effectiveness of exercise therapy in patients with osteoarthritis of the hip or knee: a systematic review. Arthritis Rheum 57:1245–1253

15. Sharma L et al (2001) The role of knee alignment in disease progression and functional decline in knee osteoarthritis. JAMA 286:188–195

16. Brouwer RW et al (2005) Braces and orthoses for treating osteoarthritis of the knee. Cochrane Database Syst Rev 25(1):CD004020

17. Kirkley A et al (1999) The effect of bracing on varus gonarthrosis. J Bone Joint Surg Am 81:539–548

18. Arnold CM, Faulkner RA (2007) The history of falls and the association of the timed up and go test to falls and near falls in older adults with hip osteoarthritis. BMC Geriatr 7:17

19. Jones A et al (2012) Impact of cane use, function, general health and energy expenditure during gait in patients with knee osteoarthritis: a randomised controlled trial. Ann Rheum Dis 71:172–179

20. McCarthy CJ et al (2006) Pulsed electromagnetic energy treatment offers no clinical benefit in reducing the pain of knee osteoarthritis: a systematic review. BMC Musculoskelet Disord 15:7–51

21. Bjordal JM et al (2007) Short-term efficacy of physical interventions in osteoarthritic knee pain. A systematic review and meta-analysis of randomised placebo-controlled trials. BMC Musculoskelet Disord 8:51

22. Manheimer E et al (2007) Meta-analysis: acupuncture for osteoarthritis of the knee. Ann Intern Med 146:868–877

23. Bjordal JM et al (2004) Non-steroidal anti-inflammatory drugs including cyclo-oxygenase-2 inhibitors, in osteo-arthritic knee pain: meta-analysis of placebo controlled trails. BMJ 329:1317–1320

24. Towheed TE et al (2006) Acetaminophen for osteoarthritis. Cochrane Database Syst Rev 1: CD004257

25. Hooper L et al (2004) The effectiveness of five strategies for the prevention of gastrointestinal toxicity induced by non-steroidal anti-inflammatory drugs: systematic review. BMJ 329:948–952

26. Kearney PM et al (2006) Do selective cyclo-oxygenase inhibitors and traditional non-steroidal anti-inflammatory drugs increase the risk of atherothrombosis ? Meta-analysis of randomised trials. BMJ 332:1302–1308

27. Schjerning Olsen AM et al (2011) Duration of treatment with nonsteroidal anti-inflammatory drugs and impact on risk of death and recurrent myocardial infarction in patients with prior myocardial infarction: a nationwide cohort study. Circulation 123:2226–2235

28. Opinion of the committee for medicinal products for human use pursuant to article 5(3) of regulation (EC) No 726/2004, for nonselective non steroidal anti-inflammatory drugs (NSAIDs)

29. Lin J et al (2005) Efficacy of topical NSAIDs in the treatment of osteoarthritis: a meta-analysis of randomized controlled trials. Chin J Evid Based Med 5(9):667–674

30. Avouac J et al (2007) Efficacy and safety of opioids for osteoarthritis: a meta-analysis of randomized controlled trials. Osteoarthritis Cartilage 15:957–965
31. Nüesch E et al (2009) Oral or transdermal opioids for osteoarthritis of the knee or hip. Cochrane Database Syst Rev 4:CD003115
32. Sawitzke AD et al (2010) Clinical efficacy and safety of glucosamine, chondroitin sulphate, their combination, celecoxib or placebo taken to treat osteoarthritis of the knee: 2-year results from GAIT. Ann Rheum Dis 69:1459–1464
33. Wandel S et al (2010) Effects of glucosamine, chondroitin, or placebo in patients with osteoarthritis of hip or knee: network meta-analysis. BMJ 341:c4675
34. Reginster JY et al (2001) Long-term effects of glucosamine sulphate on osteoarthritis progression: a randomised, placebo-controlled clinical trial. Lancet 357(9252):251–256
35. Hochberg MC (2010) Structure-modifying effects of chondroitin sulphate in knee osteoarthritis. An updated meta-analysis of randomized placebo-controlled trials of 2-year duration. Ostoarthritis Cartilage 18(suppl 1):S28–S31
36. Kahan A et al (2009) Long-term effects of chondroitins 4 and 6 sulfate on knee osteoarthritis: the study on osteoarthritis progression prevention, a two-year, randomized, double-blind, placebo-controlled trial. Arthritis Rheum 60:524–533
37. Bingham CO 3rd et al (2006) Risedronate decreases biochemical markers of cartilage degradation but does not decrease symptoms or slow radiographic progression in patients with medial compartment osteoarthritis of the knee: results of the two-year multinational knee osteoarthritis structural arthritis study. Arthritis Rheum 54(11):3494–3507
38. Neogi T et al (2008) The effect of alendronate on progression of spinal osteophytes and disc space narrowing. Ann Rheum Dis 67(10):1427–1430
39. Bruyere O et al (2008) Effects of strontium ranelate on spinal osteoarthritis progression. Ann Rheum Dis 67:335–339
40. Reginster J-Y, Badurski J, Bellamy N et al (2013) Efficacy and safety of strontium ranelate in the treatment of knee osteoarthritis: results of a double-blind, randomised placebo-controlled trial. Ann Rheum Dis 72:179–186
41. Bellamy N, Campbell J, Robinson V, Gee T, Bourne R, Wells G (2006) Intra-articular corticosteroid for treatment of osteoarthritis of the knee. Cochrane Database Syst Rev 2:CD005328
42. Navarro-Sarabia F et al (2011) A 40-month multicentre, randomised placebo-controlled study to assess the efficacy and carry-over effect of repeated intra-articular injections of hyaluronic acid in knee osteoarthritis: the AMELIA project. Ann Rheum Dis 70(11):1957–1962
43. Lane NE et al (2010) Tanezumab for the treatment of pain from osteoarthritis of the knee. N Eng J Med 363:1521–1531
44. Wood JN (2010) Nerve growth factor and pain. N Eng J Med 363:1572–1573
45. Ethgen O et al (2004) Quality of life in total hip and total knee arthroplasty: a qualitative and systematic review of the literature. J Bone Joint Surg Am 86:963–974
46. Zhang W et al (2007) OARSI recommendations for the management of hip and knee osteoarthritis, part I: critical appraisal of existing treatment guidelines and systematic review of current research evidence. Osteoarthritis Cartilage 15:981–1000
47. Soderman P et al (2001) Outcome after total hip arthroplasty: part II. Disease-specific follow-up and the Swedish National Total Hip Arthroplasty Register. Acta Orthop Scand 72:113–119
48. Rand JA et al (2003) Factors affecting the durability of primary total knee prostheses. J Bone Joint Surg Am 85:259–265
49. Katz JN (2006) Total joint replacement in osteoarthritis. Best Pract Res Clin Rheumatol 20:145–153
50. Otten R et al (2010) [Trends in the number of knee and hip arthroplasties: considerable more knee and hip prostheses due to osteoarthritis in 2030]. Ned Tijdschr Geneeskd 154:A1534
51. Griffin T et al (2007) Unicompartmental knee arthroplasty for the treatment of unicompartmental osteoarthritis: a systematic study. ANZ J Surg 77:214–221

52. Millis MB, Kim YJ (2002) Rationale for osteotomy and related procedures for hip preservation: a review. Clin Orthop Relat Res 405:108–121
53. Virolainen P, Aro HT (2004) High tibial osteotomy for the treatment of osteoarthritis of the knee: a review of the literature and a meta-analysis of follow-up studies. Arch Orthop Trauma Surg 124:258–261
54. Moseley JB et al (2002) A controlled trial of arthroscopic surgery for osteoarthritis of the knee. N Engl J Med 347(2):81–88

Part II
Functional Decline

Chapter 4
Risk Factors for Functional Decline in Osteoarthritis of the Knee or Hip

Marike van der Leeden, Cindy Veenhof, Leo D. Roorda, and Joost Dekker

Activity limitations, such as problems in walking, stair climbing, rising up, sitting down and bending down, are highly frequent in osteoarthritis (OA) of the knee or hip [1, 2]. These activity limitations may negatively affect quality of life and social participation. It has been shown that activity limitations in knee and hip OA are slowly deteriorating. In the first 3 years after diagnosis, no deterioration has been found in the OA group as a whole. Patients could either improve in their ability to perform activities, deteriorate or remain stable [3–9]. After 3 years of follow-up, deterioration of activity limitations has been observed at the level of groups of patients [6, 10–12]. However, the course of activity limitations is heterogeneous among patients. Identification of risk factors for activity limitations is therefore highly relevant [13].

Knowledge on risk factors can be used to inform patients on the likely course of their condition. Knowledge on risk factors also contributes to the understanding of mechanisms and processes, which cause activity limitations. Furthermore, risk factors are potential targets for therapeutic and preventive interventions, aiming at recovery of activities or prevention of activity limitations, respectively. This chapter provides an overview of existing knowledge from recent scientific literature on risk factors predicting the course of activity limitations in patients with OA of the knee or hip.

M. van der Leeden • L.D. Roorda
Amsterdam Rehabilitation Research Center | Reade, Amsterdam, The Netherlands

C. Veenhof
Netherlands Institute for Health Services Research (NIVEL), Utrecht, The Netherlands

J. Dekker (✉)
Department of Rehabilitation Medicine, VU University Medical Center, PO Box 7057, 1007 MB Amsterdam, The Netherlands

Department of Psychiatry, VU University Medical Center, Amsterdam, The Netherlands
e-mail: j.dekker@vumc.nl

J. Dekker (ed.), *Exercise and Physical Functioning in Osteoarthritis: Medical, Neuromuscular and Behavioral Perspectives*, Springer Briefs in Specialty Topics in Behavioral Medicine, DOI 10.1007/978-1-4614-7215-5_4, © The Author(s) 2014

Risk Factors for Activity Limitations

Various studies have sought to identify risk factors for activity limitations, or functional decline, in knee and hip OA. The order in which these risk factors are presented in this chapter is based on the International Classification of Functioning, Disability and Health (ICF). The ICF is a classification developed by the World Health Organization. The components of the ICF are as follows: body structures (the anatomic parts of the body), body functions (physiological and psychological functions of the body), activities (the execution of tasks or actions by individuals), participation (the involvement in a life situation), and environmental and personal factors (Fig. 4.1) (http://www.who.int/classification/en) [14]. Risk factors for activity limitations in knee and hip OA range from impairments in body structures (signs of joint degeneration), impairments in body functions (such as pain and muscle weakness), to personal factors (such as age and lack of physical activity).

Impairments of Body Structures

Signs of Joint Degeneration. Radiological signs that indicate joint degeneration are key findings of OA. However, the value of radiological signs to predict the course of activity limitations is unclear. There is a weak association between signs of joint degeneration on radiographs and activity limitations in cross-sectional studies [4]. Longitudinally, some studies found an association between radiological signs in the knee and future activity limitations [8, 12, 15]; however, other studies failed to find an association [4, 7, 16].

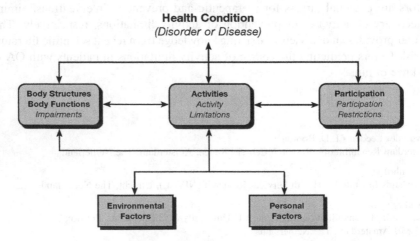

Fig. 4.1 International Classification of Functioning, Disability, and Health (ICF) (http://www. who.int/classification/en)

Impairments of Body Functions

Pain. Pain is the primary symptom of OA and appears to predict future activity limitations. The prognostic value of pain intensity in knee and hip OA was established by a systematic review of van Dijk et al.: more pain at baseline predicted more activity limitations [7]. More recent studies have confirmed this finding. In older community-dwelling adults with knee pain, pain at baseline was found to predict poor functional outcome at 18 months of follow-up [5]. Similarly, patients with knee OA (or at a high risk of knee OA) reporting less knee pain were more likely to reach a clinically relevant improvement in functional outcome over 30 months [8]. On the long term, baseline pain level appeared to a be a prognostic factor as well; Pisters et al. [9] reported higher pain at baseline to be a predictor of more activity limitations after 5 years of follow-up in patients with knee and hip OA.

Bilateral pain is likely to have a worse functional prognosis. Holla et al. found bilateral hip pain to be a predictor of activity limitations in patients with early hip OA [4]. Moreover, two other studies found bilateral pain to be a predictor of activity limitations [15, 17].

Worsening of pain has been found to have prognostic value as well, in addition to the prognostic value of pain at baseline. A study on patients with established OA of the hip or knee found that increased pain at 1-year follow-up predicts activity limitations at 3 years of follow-up [7]. In addition, in patients with nontraumatic knee symptoms (including OA) persistent knee symptoms at 1-year follow-up were associated with an unfavorable outcome, i.e., persistent knee symptoms at 6-year follow-up or having undergone knee replacement surgery [17]. These findings suggest accelerated functional decline in a subgroup of patients showing persistent or worsened pain at 1-year follow-up.

Other Symptoms. Besides pain, morning stiffness is a symptom of knee and hip OA that was found to predict functional decline [4, 15]. A longer duration of symptoms was found to be a prognostic factor in knee OA [9, 15].

Muscle Weakness. Muscle weakness has been shown to be a major risk factor for future activity limitations, especially in knee OA. Evidence from a systematic review showed that muscle weakness predicts functional decline over 3 years in individuals with knee OA [7]. This finding has been confirmed in more recent studies; greater muscle strength predicted less pain and less activity limitations at 30 months of follow-up in knee OA [18]. Similarly, patients who have or are at risk of knee OA with more knee strength were more likely to improve in their physical activities over a 30-month period [8]. Furthermore, reduction of muscle strength at 1-year follow-up predicted activity limitations at 3 years of follow-up in knee OA and baseline muscle strength predicted activity limitations at 5 years of follow-up in both knee and hip OA [7, 9].

Proprioceptive Inaccuracy, Joint Laxity, and Joint Instability. For the knee, the role of neuromuscular control in the progression of activity limitations is increasingly understood. Besides muscle weakness, laxity of the knee joint and proprioceptive inaccuracy were found to be predictors for functional decline [6]. Recent evidence suggests that instability of the knee joint affects activity limitations as well. Self-reported instability of the knee (i.e., the feeling of buckling, shifting, or giving away of the knee) contributes to activity limitations, in addition to knee pain and muscle weakness [19]. Since the impact of self-reported instability on activity limitations has so far been evaluated in cross-sectional studies only, the prognostic value of instability of the knee joint is still to be determined. It should be noted that single-leg standing balance, which may be associated to instability, predicts functional decline at 18 months of follow-up [15]. For the hip, neuromuscular factors in relation to activity limitations have hardly been studied.

Impaired Range of Joint Motion. Impaired range of motion (ROM) is a characteristic feature of OA. Although a limited number of studies are available, ROM seems to be a prognostic factor for future activity limitations in knee and hip OA. Cross-sectionally, impaired ROM was strongly associated with activity limitations [20]. In a longitudinal design, it was found that a reduction of ROM at 1-year follow-up predicted activity limitations at 3 years of follow-up in patients with established knee and hip OA [7] and baseline ROM predicted activity limitations at 5 years of follow-up in knee OA patients [9]. In addition, reduced hip flexion at baseline predicted poor 2 years outcome on activity limitations in patients with early hip OA [4].

Personal Factors

Bodyweight. Bodyweight has been found to be an important risk factor for future activity limitations, especially in knee OA. In the systematic review of van Dijk et al., bodyweight was found a risk factor in knee OA patients [6]. More recently, the evidence for bodyweight as a predictor of functional decline in knee OA has been strengthened by numerous studies [4, 5, 10, 12, 16]; only one study failed to find an association [7]. The recent systematic review by Chapple et al. confirmed bodyweight to be a predictor of both radiological progression and progression in functional decline in knee OA [21]. Thus, clear evidence exists that higher bodyweight predicts future activity limitations in knee OA. To date, there is no evidence for the role of bodyweight in the prediction of activity limitations in hip OA.

Age. Older age has been identified as a risk factor for functional decline in patients with knee OA as shown in the systematic review of van Dijk et al. [6]. Since then, results of several studies strengthened the evidence for older age as a predictor of functional decline in knee and hip OA [3, 5, 7, 9, 12]. The predictive value of age was further confirmed by the recent systematic review of Chapple et al. in knee OA [21]. In that review, it was concluded that older age is a strong predictor of both future joint degeneration and activity limitations.

Gender. Conflicting results were found regarding the association between gender and functional decline in the systematic review of van Dijk et al. [6]. In three more recent studies investigating gender as a risk factor, women were found to show more functional decline than men [3, 12, 18]. However, five other studies that investigated gender failed to find an association with functional decline [4, 5, 7, 8, 10]. Thus, the role of gender in the course of activity limitations in knee and hip OA remains unclear.

Other Sociodemographic Factors. Certain ethnic groups showed more functional decline (more decline in African-American or Hispanic-Americans compared with Whites) [3]. Furthermore, non-Western ethnicity was a predictor of poor outcome on activity limitations in early knee OA [4]. Some studies found lower educational level [6, 9, 22], lower social class and being retired [10] as risk factors for worsening of pain and activity limitations in patients with knee and hip OA, although these risk factors were not identified in other studies [4, 5, 8].

Intoxications. The prognostic value of smoking and alcohol use is unclear to date. In a study of Amin et al., men with knee OA who smoked sustained greater cartilage loss and had more severe knee pain than men who did not smoke in a 30-month period [18]. However, two other longitudinal studies that investigated smoking as a prognostic factor failed to find an association with pain and function in patients with knee and hip OA [4, 5]. The same was found for alcohol use; a single study found, surprisingly, the use of alcohol to protect against functional decline [3], whereas two other studies failed to find an association [4, 5].

Exercise and Physical Activity. Aerobic exercise was found to protect against functional decline in the systematic review of van Dijk et al. [6]. Similarly, Dunlop et al. reported that a lack of regular vigorous activity almost doubled the odds of functional decline in patients with arthritis [3]. Further support for the importance of being physically active was found by a recent study investigating the relationship between self-reported physical activity and observed functional performance in adults with knee OA. A consistent graded relationship was found between physical activity level and better performance [23]. The systematic review of Chapple et al. concluded that moderate participation in sports can be regarded safe for patients with knee OA and was not associated with progression (radiological progression as well as progression in activity limitations) [21].

Coping. A specific pain coping strategy—avoidance of activity—seems to play a role in the course of activity limitations. Avoidance refers to behavior aimed at postponing or preventing an aversive situation from occurring [24]. If physical activity causes pain, avoidance of activity postpones or prevents pain. At the short term, avoidance of activity reduces pain. However, the long-term effects of avoidance behavior can be negative. One longitudinal study found that avoidance of activity predicted a higher level of future activity limitations in patients with established knee or hip OA [9].

Self-Efficacy. Self-efficacy is defined as the conviction that one can successfully execute the behavior required to complete a task or activity [25]. Lower self-efficacy was concluded to be a predictive factor for functional decline in patients with knee OA in the systematic review of van Dijk et al. [6]. In the absence of high-quality studies, no conclusions could be drawn on the impact of self-efficacy in hip OA [6].

Psychological Distress. Various studies have investigated the role of psychological distress in functional decline. Psychological distress refers to a broad range of unpleasant mood states such as depression, anxiety, low vitality, and fatigue. Mallen et al. found that anxiety was one of the factors predicting poor functional outcome after 18 months in older patients with knee pain [5]. Depression was associated with poor functional outcome in that study as well. This last finding has also been reported by Dunlop et al., who concluded that depressive symptoms were a significant predictor of activity limitations of patients with arthritis over a 2-year period [3]. A recent study by Riddle et al. showed baseline depressive symptoms to be a statistically significant but small predictor of 2-year changes in pain and activity limitations in persons with knee pain [26]. Thus, psychological distress has been shown to have prognostic value in OA.

General Health Perception. Poorer general health perception was associated with functional decline within a 2-year follow-up period [4, 5]. Similarly, self-reported "other health problems" were associated with worsening of pain and activity limitations over a period of 7 years for both hip and knee OA [10].

Environmental Factors

Social Support. Less social support was found to predict activity limitations in patients with knee OA in the systematic review of van Dijk et al. [6]. In the absence of high-quality studies, no conclusions could be drawn on the impact of social support in hip OA.

Comorbidity

Comorbidity has been found to be a risk factor for functional decline in patients with knee and hip OA. Since comorbidity is prevalent in OA, this finding is highly relevant. Higher morbidity count predicted worsening of activity limitations in patients with both early and established OA of the knee and hip [4, 7, 9]. In a community-based sample of adults with hip and knee pain, cardiovascular morbidity and hypertension were found to be risk factors for worsening of pain and activity limitations [10]. Likewise, van Dijk et al. found cardiac disease to predict worsening of self-reported and performance-based activity limitations in patients with established hip OA [7]. Diabetes and stroke were found to be predictors of functional decline in patients with arthritis [3]. Moreover, joint pain in other joints than the hip or knee [10] or multiple-site joint pain [4, 17, 27, 28] were found to be predictors of functional decline.

Covinsky et al. demonstrated that patients with both arthritis and another chronic condition were at greater risk for developing activity limitations compared with patients with arthritis only [11]. Additionally, impairments associated with older age, i.e., cognitive and visual impairments, were found to predict functional decline [3, 7]. Despite the fact that these impairments are not intrinsically associated with OA, these findings must be taken into account in rehabilitation interventions in OA [13].

Conclusion

It can be concluded that a wide variety of risk factors for future activity limitations in knee OA (Table 4.1) and hip OA (Table 4.2) has been identified. More research on some of these factors is needed to strengthen the evidence concerning their role

Table 4.1 Risk factors for future activity limitations in OA of the knee

Risk factors	Presence of association	Evidence from
Radiological signs of joint degeneration	Unclear	>1 Longitudinal study
Pain	Yes	Systematic review
Morning stiffness	Yes	>1 Longitudinal study
Longer duration of complaints	Yes	>1 Longitudinal study
Muscle weakness	Yes	Systematic review
Proprioceptive inaccuracy	Yes	Systematic review
Laxity	Yes	Systematic review
Self-reported instability	Yes	Cross-sectional studies
Impaired range of joint motion	Yes	1 Longitudinal study
Higher bodyweight	Yes	Systematic review
Comorbidity	Yes	>1 Longitudinal study
Age	Yes	Systematic review
Gender	Unclear	1 Longitudinal study
Non-Western ethnicity	Yes	>1 Longitudinal study
Educational level	Unclear	>1 Longitudinal study
Social class	Unclear	>1 Longitudinal study
Being retired	Unclear	>1 Longitudinal study
Smoking	Unclear	>1 Longitudinal study
Alcohol use	Unclear	>1 Longitudinal study
Lower level of activity	Yes	Systematic review
Avoidance of activity	Yes	1 Longitudinal study
Lower self-efficacy	Yes	Systematic review
Psychological distress (depression and anxiety)	Yes	Systematic review
Lower general health perception	Yes	>1 Longitudinal study
Less social support	Yes	Systematic review

Table 4.2 Risk factors for future activity limitations in OA of the hip

Risk factors	Presence of association	Evidence from
Radiological signs of joint degeneration	No	>1 Longitudinal study
Pain	Yes	Systematic review
Morning stiffness	Yes	1 Longitudinal study
Longer duration of complaints	No	1 Longitudinal study
Muscle weakness	Yes	1 Longitudinal study
Proprioceptive inaccuracy		Not studied
Laxity		Not studied
Self-reported instability		Not studied
Impaired range of joint motion	Yes	>1 Longitudinal study
Higher bodyweight	No	>1 Longitudinal study
Comorbidity	Yes	>1 Longitudinal study
Age	Yes	>1 Longitudinal study
Gender	Unclear	>1 Longitudinal study
Non-Western ethnicity	No	1 Longitudinal study
Educational level	Unclear	>1 Longitudinal study
Social class	No	1 Longitudinal study
Being retired	No	1 Longitudinal study
Smoking	No	>1 Longitudinal study
Alcohol use	Unclear	>1 Longitudinal study
Lower level of activity		Not studied
Avoidance of activity	Yes	1 Longitudinal study
Lower self-efficacy		Not studied
Psychological distress (depression and anxiety)		Not studied
Lower general health perception	Yes	>1 Longitudinal study
Less social support		Not studied

in future activity limitations and to evaluate their clinical importance. Especially in hip OA, prognosis of activity limitations is difficult to date, due to a limited number of studies.

The mechanisms behind the longitudinal relationships between risk factors and activity limitations have not been explained in the present chapter. Unraveling these mechanisms is challenging and may provide new insights in targets for rehabilitation interventions. The next chapters (Chaps. 5 and 6) describe current evidence for both a neuromuscular and a behavioral model to explain activity limitations in knee and hip OA. In Chaps. 8 and 9, new insights into targets for rehabilitation interventions based on these models are given.

References

1. Lawrence RC, Felson DT, Helmick CG, Arnold LM, Choi H, Deyo RA et al (2008) Estimates of the prevalence of arthritis and other rheumatic conditions in the United States. Part II. Arthritis Rheum 58(1):26–35

2. Michaud CM, McKenna MT, Begg S, Tomijima N, Majmudar M, Bulzacchelli MT et al (2006) The burden of disease and injury in the United States 1996. Popul Health Metr 4:11
3. Dunlop DD, Semanik P, Song J, Manheim LM, Shih V, Chang RW (2005) Risk factors for functional decline in older adults with arthritis. Arthritis Rheum 52(4):1274–1282
4. Holla JF, Steultjens MP, Roorda LD, Heymans MW, Ten Wolde S, Dekker J (2010) Prognostic factors for the two-year course of activity limitations in early osteoarthritis of the hip and/or knee. Arthritis Care Res (Hoboken) 62(10):1415–1425
5. Mallen CD, Peat G, Thomas E, Lacey R, Croft P (2007) Predicting poor functional outcome in community-dwelling older adults with knee pain: prognostic value of generic indicators. Ann Rheum Dis 66(11):1456–1461
6. van Dijk GM, Dekker J, Veenhof C, van den Ende CH (2006) Course of functional status and pain in osteoarthritis of the hip or knee: a systematic review of the literature. Arthritis Rheum 55(5):779–785
7. van Dijk GM, Veenhof C, Spreeuwenberg P, Coene N, Burger BJ, van Schaardenburg D et al (2010) Prognosis of limitations in activities in osteoarthritis of the hip or knee: a three year cohort study. Arch Phys Med Rehabil 91(1):58–66
8. White DK, Keysor JJ, LaValley MP, Lewis CE, Torner JC, Nevitt MC et al (2010) Clinically important improvement in function is common in people with or at high risk of knee OA: the MOST study. J Rheumatol 37(6):1244–1251
9. Pisters MF, Veenhof C, van Dijk GM, Heymans MW, Twisk JWR, Dekker J et al (2012) The course of limitations in activities over five years in patients with knee and hip osteoarthritis: risk factors for future functional decline. Osteoarthritis Cartilage 20(6):503–510
10. Peters TJ, Sanders C, Dieppe P, Donovan J (2005) Factors associated with change in pain and disability over time: a community-based prospective observational study of hip and knee osteoarthritis. Br J Gen Pract 55(512):205–211
11. Covinsky KE, Lindquist K, Dunlop DD, Gill TM, Yelin E (2008) Effect of arthritis in middle age on older-age functioning. J Am Geriatr Soc 56(1):23–28
12. Roos EM, Bremander AB, Englund M, Lohmander LS (2008) Change in self-reported outcomes and objective physical function over 7 years in middle-aged subjects with or at high risk of knee osteoarthritis. Ann Rheum Dis 67(4):505–510
13. Dekker J, van Dijk GM, Veenhof C (2009) Risk factors for functional decline in osteoarthritis of the hip or knee. Curr Opin Rheumatol 21(5):520–524
14. Stucki G, Cieza A, Melvin J (2007) The International Classification of Functioning, Disability and Health (ICF): a unifying model for the conceptual description of the rehabilitation strategy. J Rehabil Med 39(4):279–285
15. Thomas E, Peat G, Mallen C, Wood L, Lacey R, Duncan R et al (2008) Predicting the course of functional limitation among older adults with knee pain: do local signs, symptoms and radiographs add anything to general indicators? Ann Rheum Dis 67(10):1390–1398
16. Paradowski PT, Englund M, Lohmander LS, Roos EM (2005) The effect of patient characteristics on variability in pain and function over two years in early knee osteoarthritis. Health Qual Life Outcomes 3:59
17. Kastelein M, Luijsterburg PA, Belo JN, Verhaar JA, Koes BW, Bierma-Zeinstra SM (2011) Six-year course and prognosis of nontraumatic knee symptoms in adults in general practice: a prospective cohort study. Arthritis Care Res (Hoboken) 63(9):1287–1294
18. Amin S, Niu J, Guermazi A, Grigoryan M, Hunter DJ, Clancy M et al (2007) Cigarette smoking and the risk for cartilage loss and knee pain in men with knee osteoarthritis. Ann Rheum Dis 66(1):18–22
19. van der Esch M, Knoop J, van der Leeden M, Voorneman R, Gerritsen M, Reiding D et al (2012) Self-reported knee instability and activity limitations in patients with knee osteoarthritis: results from the AMS-OA cohort. Clin Rheumatol 31(10):1505–1510, Ref type: Abstract

20. Steultjens MP, Dekker J, van Baar ME, Oostendorp RA, Bijlsma JW (2000) Range of joint motion and disability in patients with osteoarthritis of the knee or hip. Rheumatology (Oxford) 39(9):955–961
21. Chapple CM, Nicholson H, Baxter GD, Abbott JH (2011) Patient characteristics that predict progression of knee osteoarthritis: a systematic review of prognostic studies. Arthritis Care Res (Hoboken) 63(8):1115–1125
22. Juhakoski R, Tenhonen S, Anttonen T, Kauppinen T, Arokoski JP (2008) Factors affecting self-reported pain and physical function in patients with hip osteoarthritis. Arch Phys Med Rehabil 89(6):1066–1073
23. Dunlop DD, Song J, Semanik PA, Sharma L, Chang RW (2011) Physical activity levels and functional performance in the osteoarthritis initiative: a graded relationship. Arthritis Rheum 63(1):127–136
24. Leeuw M, Goossens ME, Linton SJ, Crombez G, Boersma K, Vlaeyen JW (2007) The fear-avoidance model of musculoskeletal pain: current state of scientific evidence. J Behav Med 30(1):77–94
25. Harrison AL (2004) The influence of pathology, pain, balance, and self-efficacy on function in women with osteoarthritis of the knee. Phys Ther 84(9):822–831
26. Riddle DL, Kong X, Fitzgerald GK (2011) Psychological health impact on 2-year changes in pain and function in persons with knee pain: data from the Osteoarthritis Initiative. Osteoarthritis Cartilage 19(9):1095–1101
27. Belo JN, Berger MY, Koes BW, Bierma-Zeinstra SM (2009) Prognostic factors in adults with knee pain in general practice. Arthritis Rheum 61(2):143–151
28. Peat G, Thomas E, Wilkie R, Croft P (2006) Multiple joint pain and lower extremity disability in middle and old age. Disabil Rehabil 28(24):1543–1549

Chapter 5
Neuromuscular Mechanisms Explaining Functional Decline

Martin van der Esch and Joost Dekker

Activity limitations are one of the main consequences of knee osteoarthritis (OA) [1–4]. For knee OA, limitations during daily activities are primarily related to walking, stair climbing, and transfers (such as rising up from or sitting down on a chair, rising up from a bed, and getting into and out of a car) [1]. Activity limitations are already present early in the disease process and progress over time [3]. Risk factors for activity limitations in patients with knee OA are described in Chap. 4. Neuromuscular risk factors, including poor muscle strength, decreased joint proprioception, joint laxity, and high varus–valgus motion, are clinically well-accepted risk factors for activity limitations [4–8]. In an attempt to gain insight into the relationship between risk factors and activity limitations in patients with knee OA, a neuromuscular model has recently been presented [4]. Poor muscle strength has been shown to be one of the strongest risk factors for activity limitations [4]. Additionally, poor proprioception (inaccurate proprioceptive acuity), high knee laxity, and high varus–valgus motion may also be associated with activity limitations, although the knowledge of these aspects of the neuromuscular model is sparse.

This chapter describes the neuromuscular model and reviews some aspects of the neuromuscular model in relation to activity limitations in knee OA patients, namely by outlining the procedures used for evaluating the model and, by presenting the current scientific evidence for components of the model: muscle strength, joint proprioception, joint laxity, and varus–valgus motion.

M. van der Esch
Amsterdam Rehabilitation Research Center | Reade, Amsterdam, The Netherlands

J. Dekker (✉)
Department of Rehabilitation Medicine, VU University Medical Center, PO Box 7057, 1007 MB Amsterdam, The Netherlands

Department of Psychiatry, VU University Medical Center, Amsterdam, The Netherlands
e-mail: j.dekker@vumc.nl

J. Dekker (ed.), *Exercise and Physical Functioning in Osteoarthritis: Medical, Neuromuscular and Behavioral Perspectives*, Springer Briefs in Specialty Topics in Behavioral Medicine, DOI 10.1007/978-1-4614-7215-5_5, © The Author(s) 2014

The Neuromuscular Model

When performing daily activities, such as walking, stair climbing, and rising up from or sitting down on a chair, external and internal load changes affecting the knee need to be accommodated. An accurate neuromuscular system accommodates these loads. The knee joint's behavior during the performance of daily activities is influenced by several factors including muscle strength, proprioceptive acuity, joint laxity, and varus–valgus motion. These factors determine to what extent a state of equilibrium of the knee joint (i.e., stability of the knee joint) can be maintained.

Muscle weakness is a crucial factor in the explanation of activity limitations in OA [4]. Muscle weakness is thought to have a *direct* impact on activity limitations; muscle strength is required for the adequate performance of activities. Muscle weakness may also have an *indirect* impact on the performance of activities, through instability of the knee joint. Muscle weakness may cause instability of the knee thereby leading to activity limitations.

In addition to muscle weakness, poor proprioception is thought to contribute to instability of the knee joint as well. Proprioception is impaired in knee OA [9]. It is hypothesized that poor proprioception aggravates the impact of muscle weakness on instability of the knee and thereby on activity limitations.

Joint laxity may contribute to instability of the knee joint. Laxity of the joint is due to impairment of the passive restraint system of the joint (primarily the ligaments and the capsule). Stronger muscles may compensate the impact of laxity on instability. Conversely, the impact of muscle weakness on instability and activity limitations is hypothesized to be aggravated by joint laxity; muscle weakness in combination with laxity has a strong impact on activity limitations.

Finally, high varus–valgus motion of the knee joint during walking may also contribute to instability of the knee joint. A high motion in the frontal plane in the weight acceptance and midstance phases of walking may be compensated by muscle strength. It is hypothesized that high varus–valgus motion aggravates the impact of muscle strength on knee instability and thereby on activity limitations.

The neuromuscular model offers an explanation of how muscle weakness, poor proprioception, joint laxity, and high varus–valgus motion are involved in generating limitations of daily activities in patients with knee OA. As shown in Fig. 5.1, the model hypothesizes the direct relationship between muscle weakness and activity limitations, as well as the combined influence of muscle weakness and poor proprioception, and muscle weakness and high laxity, and muscle weakness and high varus–valgus motion on activity limitations.

Neuromuscular model

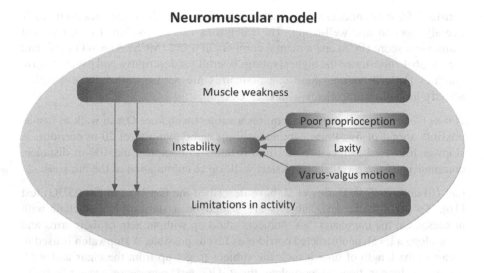

Fig. 5.1 Neuromuscular factors and activity limitations

Measurement of Activity Limitations and Neuromuscular Factors

Activity Limitations

Both in clinical practice and in scientific research on patients with knee OA, activity limitations as outcome are evaluated using various instruments. Activity limitations are defined as difficulties an individual may have in executing daily activities [10, 11]. The Outcome Measures in Rheumatology Trials (OMERACT) group defined a core set of outcome dimensions for clinical studies, which are pain, physical function (the performance of daily activities), and patients global assessment [12]. In line with these outcome dimensions, activity limitations of knee OA patients are usually assessed with self-report questionnaires [Western Ontario and McMaster Universities Osteoarthritis Index (WOMAC) physical function subscale and the SF-36 physical function subscale] and with performance-based timed tests (walk test, GUG, and stair climb) [12].

WOMAC and SF-36. The WOMAC is a disease-specific measure of pain, stiffness, and physical function for individuals with OA of the knee [13, 14]. The WOMAC, with a possible range of 0–96, includes 5 items related to pain, 2 items related to stiffness, and 17 items related to physical function (PF). Each item is scored on a 5-point Likert scale. Reliability and validity of the WOMAC have been established [13]. Higher scores on the WOMAC represent greater limitations in function. The ICC for Dutch WOMAC physical functioning was 0.92 [13]. The Medical Outcome Study 36-Item Short Form-36 (SF-36) is a generic questionnaire [15]. The SF-36 consists of a series of questions, which are divided into eight categories rating their overall function and well-being. The categories can be combined to a physical component score (PCS) and a mental component score (MCS). The WOMAC and the SF-36 demonstrated the highest ratings overall for descriptive and psychometric qualities [12]. Therefore, these questionnaires are recommended for evaluating activity limitations in patients with knee OA.

100-m Walk Test. This walk test requires a subject with knee OA to walk as fast as possible a total of five times continuously up and down a level 20-m corridor. A stopwatch is used to measure the time it takes to complete the 100-m distance, commencing from a verbal cue to start walking to culmination of the 5th pass.

Get Up and Go Test. Hurley et al. have described the Get Up and Go (GUG) test [16]. To perform the test, subjects are seated on a standard-height chair with armrests. On the command "go" subjects stand up without help of their arms and walk along a level, unobstructed corridor as fast as possible. A stopwatch is used to measure the length of time it took the subject to get up from the chair and walk 15 m. A longer time to complete the GUG test represents greater activity limitations. The intraclass correlation coefficients (ICCs) for the intratester and the intertester reliability were both 0.98 [17].

Stair-Climb Test. To perform the stair-climb test subjects stand at the foot of a stairway comprising several steps (e.g., 12 steps with a 16-cm high), and on the command "go", ascend the stairs as fast as possible. After a period of rest at the top of the stairs, subjects descend the stairs as fast as possible. A stopwatch is used for timing. The correlation between the time of step ascent and descent was $r = 0.90$ (95 %CI 0.85–0.97) [18].

Muscle Strength

In many studies, knee extension and flexion strength has been assessed isokinetically with a dynamometer [5–8]. Various instruments for isokinetic assessment of muscle strength are available; an example is given in Fig. 5.2. According to a standardized protocol, patients are usually sitting on a bench and secured to the testing device with chest, pelvis, and thigh straps. Furthermore, the measurement is standardized for the position of the ankle pad and the position of the knee opposite to the mechanical axis of the dynamometer. In general, during testing, the range of knee motion is limited to 20–80° for knee joint protection. Usually, patients perform submaximal contractions as a warm-up period, building up to maximal contractions. Patients perform a series of maximal test repetitions with right–left order of testing usually alternated between patients. The maximum score of the three repetitions is mostly used. At least two methods are used in analyses. The mean of extension and flexion strength of each leg is computed to obtain mean muscle strength, or the maximum of one of the measurements is used. Subsequently, mean muscle strength in Nm is divided by the patient's body weight.

Fig. 5.2 The assessment of isokinetic extension and flexion muscle strength

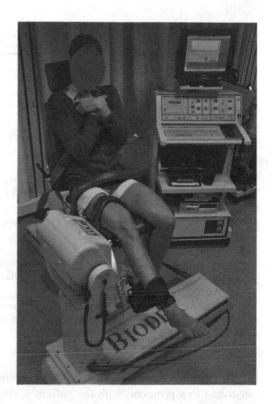

In other OA studies, muscle strength has been tested isometrically by using a simple hand-held dynamometer [19, 20]. In the clinic, a hand-held dynamometer gives the opportunity to measure muscle strength in a feasible way, when dynamometers for isokinetically measurements are not available.

Knee Proprioception

Knee proprioception has been defined as the conscious and/or unconscious perception of position and movement of an extremity or a joint in space [9]. The perception of proprioception partially derives from integrated afferent neural input arising from mechanoreceptors in different structures of the knee (joint capsule and ligaments, muscles, tendons, and associated tissue) but is also influenced by afferents from outside the knee (vestibular organ, visual system, and cutaneous and proprioceptive receptors from other body parts). Table 5.1 gives an overview of mechanoreceptors of the knee, their location, and the stimulus specificity.

Proprioceptive acuity of the knee can be assessed by the detection of joint motion or joint position [7, 9, 21–32]. For both measurements, a multicomponent device measures angular displacement of the knee joint in a nonweight-bearing position. Visual and auditory stimuli, mechanical vibrations, cutaneous tension, and pressure cues should be minimized during assessment.

Table 5.1 Proprioceptive receptors of the knee

Receptor	Location	Stimulus specificity
Active receptors		
Muscle spindles	Muscles fibers	Muscle elongation, velocity, and acceleration (especially at mid-range of knee angle)
Golgi tendon organs	Tendons	Force developed by the muscle
Articular mechanoreceptors		
Pacinian corpuscles (quick-adapting receptors)	Ligaments, menisci, capsule	Small (dynamic) changes in tissue deformation
Ruffini endings (slow-adapting receptors)	Ligaments, menisci, capsule	Joint angle (especially at extreme knee angles), velocity, intra-articular pressure, and strains
Golgi receptors	Ligaments, menisci, capsule	Joint angle (especially at extreme knee angles)
Bare nerve endings	Various tissues in and around knee	(Excessive) tissue deformation, pain, inflammation

Source: Knoop J, Steultjens MP, van der Leeden M, van der Esch M, Thorstensson CA, Roorda LD et al. Proprioception in knee osteoarthritis: a narrative review. Osteoarthritis Cartilage 2011; 19:381–388. Reprinted with permission

The measurement of knee joint movement and position is conducted according to a protocol, with the patient seated in a chair (Fig. 5.3). The sitting position creates an optimum positioning as the axis of rotation of the tibiofemoral joint can be aligned with the axis of rotation of the device. An ankle cuff should be used to minimize extraneous movements. To eliminate any contribution from cutaneous receptors and to avoid skin contact with clothing and the lever arm, the lower leg is placed on a freely moving footrest. Patients should be given standard instructions, informing them that the right or left leg will be tested in a random order.

For measuring joint movement sense both legs are moved to a starting position and after stopping the movement a random delay occurs before motion onset. Following this delay, a computer-controlled constant angular motion of one knee is initiated. The patient pushes a button after definite detection of knee joint movement. The threshold for detection of knee joint movement is defined as the difference, in degrees, between the actual onset of motion and the patient's detection of knee joint motion [7, 31]. A large difference between the actual onset of motion and the patient's detection expresses poor proprioception.

For measuring joint position sense, one knee is moved from a starting position to a testing position [25]. Following a delay, the knee is returned to the starting position. From that position the knee is extended to the original testing position and the patient has to detect when this position has been reached. The angular displacement between the test position and the perceived position is recorded. The threshold for detection of knee joint position is defined as the difference, in degrees,

Fig. 5.3 The assessment of
joint motion sense and joint
position sense

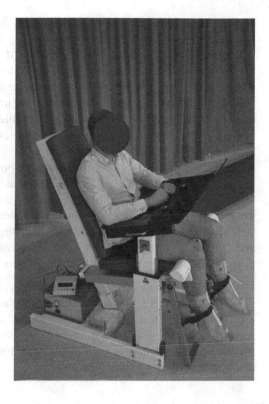

between the actual onset of the position and the patient's detection of the knee joint
position. A large difference between the original onset of position and the patient's
detection expresses poor proprioception.

At least two methods are used in analyses. The mean of three measurements of
each knee are computed to obtain mean knee joint movement and knee joint
position, respectively. Alternatively, the maximum of one of the measurements of
knee joint movement and knee joint position is used. ICCs for intrarater reliability
for the assessment of patients with OA and patients without OA by a single experienced tester were 0.91 and 0.87 for joint movement detection, respectively [31].

Alternative Measures of Knee Proprioception

Shortly, two alternative methods of measuring knee proprioception will be
described: measuring joint position sense with an electrogoniometer and measuring
the vibratory perception threshold.

Electrogoniometer. In several studies, a twin-axis electrogoniometer has been used
for measuring knee joint position sense [24, 30, 32–34]. The electrogoniometer

has been attached to the outside of the leg [24, 30]. The electrogoniometer is mostly attached to the lateral aspect of the lower leg using adhesive (double sided) tape with the lower sensor just below the head of the fibula (in line with the lateral malleolus) and the upper sensor taped at the top of the lateral femoral condyle, in line with the great trochanter. The goniometer is connected to a hand-held display unit that will give a continuous, real-time digital reading of the flexion angle. It is recommended that patients are sitting on a table with knees and hips at 90° flexion and the knees hanging over the edge of a table, the axis of rotation aligned with the tibiofemoral joint's axis of rotation.

Measurements in weight-bearing standing positions have been reported too, with the aim to measure joint position sense in a functional way [34]. However, the influence of different afferent systems as the vestibular system, muscle strength and the proprioception of other joints may influence the outcome of this assessment.

The outcome of the test is the difference in degrees between the perceived position and the actual test position. A large difference between the detected test joint position and the original test position expresses decreased proprioceptive acuity.

Vibratory Perception Measurement. Recently, it was found that vibratory perception threshold (VPT) is reduced in knee OA patients [35, 36]. Vibratory perception travels through similar neurologic pathways as the afferents for proprioception; therefore, vibratory sense may also be decreased in knee OA. VPT is a sensory measure that is commonly used to evaluate diabetic neuropathy and that has been associated with neuropathic arthropathy.

Knee Laxity

Joint laxity has been defined as the displacement or rotation of the tibia with respect to the femur in the varus–valgus direction [37–40]. The inside and outside displacement of the tibia reflects the capsule-ligamentous stretch when load is applied to the knee joint. The total displacement depends on the stretch capability of the ligaments, capsule, and other soft tissues.

Varus–valgus laxity can be measured using a device that provides thigh and lower leg immobilization, a stable knee angle in flexion of 20°, and fixed varus and valgus load [39, 40]. An example of a device is presented (Fig. 5.4). Laxity is measured (in degrees) as the movement in the frontal plane after varus and valgus load. In several studies, a weight of 1.12 kg has been used to load the lower leg [6]. This load can be applied to the lower leg both medially and laterally, resulting in varus or valgus movement in the knee joint.

It is recommended that all measurements of laxity are performed in adherence to a protocol, including the use of anatomic landmarks for patient positioning, patient instructions, and the examiner's position. Right–left order of testing is alternated between patients. In analyses, the mean in degrees for laxity of the right and left knees obtained from several measurements is mostly used or the

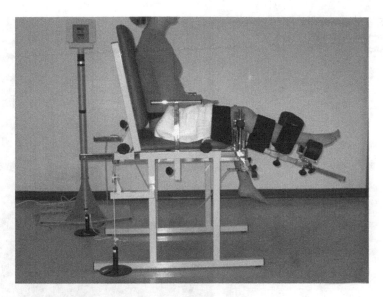

Fig. 5.4 The assessment of varus–valgus laxity of the knee

maximum of one of the measurements. The ICC for intra- and interrater reliability of the measurements in healthy persons was 0.80 and 0.88, respectively [39].

Knee Varus–Valgus Motion. Knee varus–valgus motion has been defined as the movement in the frontal plane during the weight acceptance phase and the midstance phase of walking [8]. Varus–valgus motion has been measured by a motion analyses system to record 3D position of light-emitting diode markers (see Fig. 5.5). Synchronously, 3D ground reaction force can be recorded by using a force plate. Finally, with MATLAB software, the anatomical axes, the 3D motion, and the loading data can be reconstructed. Using this software, the ground reaction force curve represents itself as an M shape, from which the loading response phase (i.e., from zero to the first peak) and midstance (i.e., the lowest point of the M shape in between two peaks) can be determined. These two parts of the ground reaction force curve can be used to determine (1) the knee varus–valgus range of motion (VV-ROM) and (2) the varus–valgus position (VVP). The difference between the peak excursion in varus direction and the peak excursion in valgus direction reflects VV-ROM (in degrees). VVP is the position of the knee in midstance. VVP (in degrees) can be obtained by comparing the position of the knee in the varus or valgus direction in midstance with the position of the knee at the start of measurement (anatomical posture, prior to walking).

In order to measure VV-ROM and VVP, subjects are instructed to walk at a self-selected speed along a walkway. The mean in degrees for VV-ROM and VVP of the right and left knees obtained from at least three measurements can be used for analysis.

Fig. 5.5 The assessment of varus–valgus motion of the knee

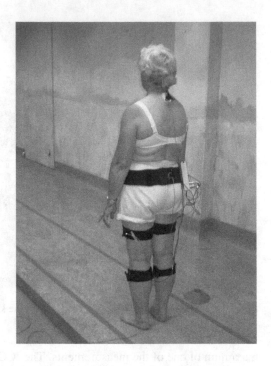

Integration of Neuromuscular Factors: Knee Joint Stability

In stabilizing the knee joint, all four factors of the neuromuscular model are involved to maintain a position of the knee or to control the movements of the knee under differing external loads. Knee stability is a key component of the mechanical environment of the normal knee joint. In an unloaded state, the ligaments, capsule, and other soft tissues provide static knee stability. Under loaded conditions, dynamic stability of the knee is provided by muscle strength, proprioceptive acuity, and minimal varus–valgus motion. The processing of proprioceptive input by the central nervous system results in the contraction of periarticular muscles, which reduces unexpected and sudden variability in knee motions and therefore stabilizes the knee.

Dynamic knee joint stability and variability in knee motion can be measured during treadmill walking [42]. Yakhdani et al. [41] used the Lyapunov exponent to quantify sagittal knee stability in a group of knee OA patients. The Lyapunov exponent quantifies the effect of corrections to small perturbations during walking [42]. In other words, this is the degree to which kinematics of walking remain the same over time. This is a relatively new measure of stability. Further research is needed to demonstrate its value as a measure of stability in knee OA.

Self-Reported Knee Instability. When the knee is not able to maintain a position or when movements are not controlled, patients may report the perception of knee instability, described as a perception of slipping, buckling, or giving way of the knee [43]. The perception of slipping refers to a smoothly gave way feeling. Bucking refers to a sudden and full gave way perception of the knee. Both perceptions indicate that the knee is not under neuromuscular control during daily activities. Approximately, two-thirds of patients with knee OA report knee instability [18, 43–45].

Self-reported knee instability might be assessed with the question to what degree the perception of instability affects daily activities, according to the study of Fitzgerald et al. [44]. Another way of questioning is by asking the presence or absence of the perception of instability, without the relationship with daily activities [18, 43–45]. The perception of instability might be assessed by the question: "Have you had an episode in the past 3 months where your knee slipped (partial gave way) or buckled (total gave way)?" Persons who answered "yes" on one of the two questions are asked to indicate which knee gave way and how many times in the past 3 months, they had had such an episode. Additionally, it can be asked what they were doing when their knee gave way. Options are different aspects of activity limitations such as walking, descending or ascending stairs, twisting or turning, or other.

Scientific Evidence for the Neuromuscular Model

Several studies have focused on the components of the neuromuscular model in an attempt to validate the model [4, 6–8]. In these studies, the impact of muscle weakness as well as decreased proprioceptive acuity, joint laxity, and high varus–valgus motion was assessed. It was shown that muscle weakness is the most important component of the model and thereby the determinant of activity limitations. However, the impact of muscle weakness on activity limitations is influenced by knee joint proprioceptive acuity, knee laxity, and high varus–valgus motion.

Muscle Weakness and Activity Limitations

Muscle weakness is an important characteristic in knee OA and a frequent finding in knee OA patients [5–8, 33, 46–51]. Between knee OA patients, there is a high variability in muscle strength ranging from normal muscle strength to severe muscle weakness [48]. Muscle weakness is a risk factor for knee OA onset, progression, poor clinical outcome, and activity limitations [4, 5, 46, 47, 51, 52]. In a cross-sectional study by Slemenda et al., the quadriceps muscle was found on average 20 % weaker among those with radiographic signs of OA [49]. Steultjens et al. [48] showed that muscle weakness in knee OA patients accounted for 15–20 % of activity limitations related to the lower extremity. Recently, an association between muscle strength and activity limitations was found in early knee OA patients, indicating a higher level of activity limitations in participants with weaker muscles [52]. These findings confirm the premise that muscle weakness is an important risk factor for activity limitations in early and established knee OA patients.

Knee Joint Proprioception and Activity Limitations

A recent narrative review [9] has shown that proprioceptive accuracy is related to activity limitations in knee OA patients. Knee proprioceptive acuity is presumed to be required for stability of the knee during static posture and coordination of movements. Poor proprioceptive acuity is related to activity limitations in two ways: directly and indirectly. A direct relationship has been demonstrated; however, that relationship was rather weak [5, 7]. An indirect relationship between proprioceptive acuity and activity limitations was also shown [7]. Poor proprioceptive acuity aggravated the impact of muscle weakness on activity limitations. This means that in the presence of poor proprioceptive acuity, muscle weakness results in more activity limitations compared to a situation with muscle weakness and adequate proprioceptive acuity (see Fig. 5.6a–c). This observation was made using walking and GUG time; on the WOMAC-pf score, the pattern was the same, but it was not statistically significant. Thus, in knee OA patients with an inadequate neuromuscular system, due to a poor proprioceptive acuity, activities such as walking are more affected by muscle weakness than in knee OA patients with an adequate neuromuscular system.

The relationship between knee joint proprioceptive acuity and activity limitations has been demonstrated in other cross-sectional studies too [5, 24]. A modest relationship has also been found in a longitudinal study, showing that the increase in activity limitations in time was higher in patients with poor proprioception than in patients with accurate proprioception [30]. Sharma et al. [27] described that proprioceptive acuity is a more generalized process and that a change in proprioceptive acuity was not only related to the affected side or joints but also to the unaffected side. Knee proprioceptive acuity may be not a local joint process, but a more systemic process, which is generalized over several joints; however, the evidence for this generalization process is weak. More studies on proprioception are needed in knee OA patients to explore the role of proprioceptive acuity deficits as a generalized process, and its relationship to activity limitations longitudinally.

Knee Joint Laxity and Activity Limitations

Knee joint laxity refers to the behavior of the joint during passive varus–valgus rotation and is presumed to be the static component of knee joint stability. High knee joint laxity is related to activity limitations indirectly; high laxity aggravated the impact of muscle weakness on activity limitations [6]; in knees with high laxity,

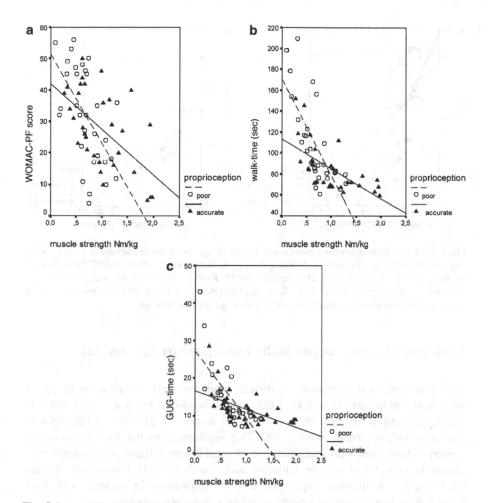

Fig. 5.6 (a–c) The relationship between activity limitations and muscle strength in an accurate proprioception (low JMDT <4.3°) group and a poor proprioception (high JMDT >4.3°) group. (a) Walking time vs. muscle strength. (b) GUG time vs. muscle strength. (c) WOMAC-PF vs. muscle strength. *JMDT* Joint Motion Detection Threshold (degrees). *Source*: Van der Esch M, Steultjens M, Harlaar J, Knol D, Lems W, Dekker J. Joint proprioception, muscle strength, and functional ability in patients with osteoarthritis of the knee. Arthritis Rheum 2007; 57:787–793. Reprinted with permission

muscle weakness was stronger associated with activity limitations than in patients with low laxity, see Fig. 5.7. By way of explanation, it was hypothesized that in highly lax knees, the loss of static stability is compensated by higher coactivation of knee muscles. This means that less muscle strength is available for the execution of daily activities [6]. As a result, knee OA patients with high laxity of the knee joint are more at risk for developing activity limitations in the presence of muscle weakness.

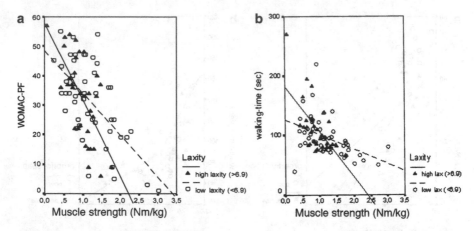

Fig. 5.7 (**a, b**) The relationship between activity limitations and muscle strength in a low (<6.9°) and a high (>6.9°) laxity group. (**a**) Walking time vs. muscle strength. (**b**) WOMAC-PF vs. muscle strength. *Source*: Van der Esch M, Steultjens MPM, Knol D, Dinant H, Dekker J. Joint laxity modifies the relationship between muscle strength and disability in patients with osteoarthritis of the knee. Arthritis Rheum 2006;55:953–959. Reprinted with permission

Knee Joint Varus–Valgus Motion and Activity Limitations

Knee joint varus–valgus motion is indirectly related to activity limitations [8, 53]. It was found that in patients with knee OA, muscle weakness has a stronger impact on activity limitations when the knee varus–valgus motion is higher than in patients with low varus–valgus motion (see Fig. 5.8). This result suggests that high varus–valgus motion is associated with inefficient use of muscle strength and that patients need greater magnitudes of muscle activities during walking [54]. Conversely, muscle weakness has a stronger impact on activity limitations in patients with high varus–valgus motion than in patients with low varus–valgus motion.

Knee Stability

Muscle weakness, poor proprioception, joint laxity, and high varus–valgus motion are hypothesized to cause instability of the knee joint and thereby activity limitations. These variables should be interpreted as components of knee stability, but they are not direct measures of knee instability. Few studies have attempted to assess instability of the knee joint directly [41, 42]. Yakhdani et al. assessed dynamic instability using the Lyapunov exponent [41]. Further research is needed to evaluate whether this is a valid measure of knee instability in OA. Another indirect measurement of knee instability is the measurement of the perception of giving way of the knee by self-report. Four studies have dealt with the self-reported

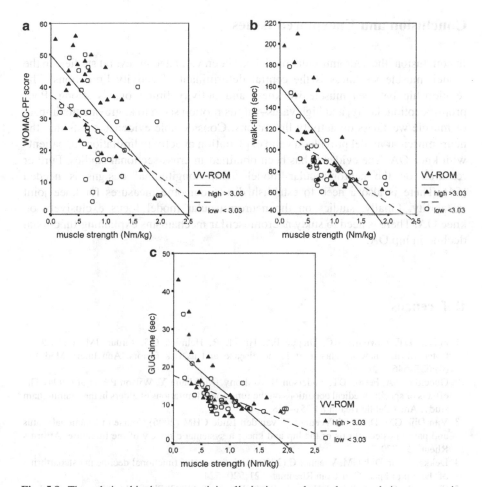

Fig. 5.8 The relationship between activity limitations and muscle strength in an excessive VV-ROM (>3.03°) group and a minimal VV-ROM (<3.03°) group in the loading response phase of the gait cycle. (**a**) walking time vs. muscle strength. (**b**) GUG time vs. muscle strength. (**c**) WOMAC-PF vs. muscle strength. *Source*: Van der Esch M, Steultjens M, Harlaar J, et al. Varus-valgus motion and functional ability in patients with knee osteoarthritis. Ann Rheum Dis 2008;67:471–477. Reprinted with permission

knee instability and activity limitations [18, 43–46]. These studies concluded that self-reported knee instability and activity limitations are related. Recently, Knoop et al. found that muscle weakness was strongly related to self-reported knee instability, while knee joint proprioception and knee laxity were not [45]. This may indicate that muscle strength is a dominant variable related to the perception of knee instability. Possibly, the effects of poor proprioception, laxity, and high varus–valgus motion are rather small compared to the effect of muscle strength, and therefore too small to influence self-reported instability.

Conclusion and Unexplored Issues

In conclusion, the neuromuscular model has been validated in several studies. In the model, muscle weakness is the central determinant of activity limitations. The relationship between muscle weakness and activity limitations is strong. Poor proprioception, laxity, and high varus–valgus motion seem to aggravate the impact of muscle weakness on activity limitations. Considerable evidence exists that the neuromuscular model provides a valid explanation of activity limitations in patients with knee OA. The evidence has been obtained in cross-sectional studies. Further research on the neuromuscular model using longitudinal designs is needed [54]. There is also a need to establish direct outcome measures for knee joint instability. Finally, studies on the neuromuscular model focus exclusively on knee OA. There is need to study neuromuscular mechanisms explaining functional decline in hip OA.

References

1. Felson DT, Lawrence RC, Dieppe PA, Hirsch R, Helmick CG, Jordan JM et al (2000) Osteoarthritis: new insights. Part 1: the disease and its risk factors. Ann Intern Med 133 (8):635–646
2. Guccione AA, Felson DT, Anderson JJ, Anthony JM, Zhang Y, Wilson PW et al (1994) The effects of specific medical conditions on the functional limitations of elders in the Framingham study. Am J Public Health 84:351–358
3. Van Dijk GM, Dekker J, Veenhof C, van den Ende CHM (2006) Course of functional status and pain in osteoarthritis of the hip and knee: a systematic review of the literature. Arthritis Rheum 55:779–785
4. Dekker J, van Dijk GM, Veenhof C (2009) Risk factors for functional decline in osteoarthritis of the hip or knee. Curr Opin Rheumatol 21:520–524
5. Sharma L, Cahue S, Song J, Hayes K, Pai Y, Dunlop D (2003) Physical functioning over three years in knee osteoarthritis. Arthritis Rheum 48:3359–3370
6. Van der Esch M, Steultjens MPM, Knol D, Dinant H, Dekker J (2006) Joint laxity modifies the relationship between muscle strength and disability in patients with osteoarthritis of the knee. Arthritis Rheum 55:953–959
7. Van der Esch M, Steultjens M, Harlaar J, Knol D, Lems W, Dekker J (2007) Joint propriocep-tion, muscle strength, and functional ability in patients with osteoarthritis of the knee. Arthritis Rheum 57:787–793
8. Van der Esch M, Steultjens M, Harlaar J et al (2008) Varus-valgus motion and functional ability in patients with knee osteoarthritis. Ann Rheum Dis 67:471–477
9. Knoop J, Steultjens MP, van der Leeden M, van der Esch M, Thorstensson CA, Roorda LD et al (2011) Proprioception in knee osteoarthritis: a narrative review. Osteoarthritis Cartilage 19:381–388
10. World Health Organization (2002) Towards a common language for functioning, disability and health: ICF. WHO, Geneva
11. Botha-Scheepers S, Riyazi N, Kroon HM, Scharloo M, Houwing-Duistermaat JJ, Slagboom E, Rosendaal FR, Breedveld FC, Kloppenburg M (2006) Activity limitations in the lower extremities in patients with osteoarthritis: the modifying effects of illness perceptions and mental health. Osteoarthritis Cartilage 14(11):1104–1110

12. Veenhof C, Bijlsma JW, van den Ende CH, van Dijk GM, Pisters MF, Dekker J (2006) Psychometric evaluation of osteoarthritis questionnaires: a systematic review of the literature. Arthritis Rheum 55:480–492
13. Roorda L, Jones C, Waltz M, Lankhorst G, Bouter L, van der IJken J, Willems W, Heyligers I, Voaklander D, Kelly K, Suarez-Almazor M (2004) Satisfactory cross cultural equivalence of the Dutch WOMAC in patients with hip osteoarthritis waiting for arthroplasty. Ann Rheum Dis 63:36–42
14. Bellamy N, Buchanan WW, Goldsmith CH, Campbell J, Stitt LW (1988) Validation study of WOMAC: a health status instrument for measuring clinically important patient relevant outcomes to antirheumatic drug therapy in patients with osteoarthritis of the hip or knee. J Rheumatol 15:1833–1840
15. Ware JE Jr, Keller SD, Hatoum HT, Kong SX (1999) The SF-36 Arthritis-Specific Health Index (ASHI): I. Development and cross-validation of scoring algorithms. Med Care 37 (5 Suppl):MS40–MS50
16. Hurley MV, Scott DL, Rees J, Newham DJ (1997) Sensorimotor changes and functional performance in patients with knee osteoarthritis. Ann Rheum Dis 56:641–648
17. Piva SR, Fitzgerald GK, Irrgang JJ, Bouzubar F, Starz TW (2004) Get up and go test in patients with knee osteoarthritis. Arch Phys Med Rehabil 85:284–289
18. van der Esch M, Knoop J, van der Leeden M, Voorneman R, Gerritsen M, Reiding D, Romviel S, Knol D, Lems W, Dekker J, Roorda L (2012) Self-reported knee instability and activity limitations in patients with knee osteoarthritis: results from the AMS-OA cohort. Cin Rheumatol 31:1505–1510
19. Carpenter MR, Carpenter RL, Peel J, Zukley LM, Angelopoulou KM, Fischer I, Angelopoulos TJ, Rippe JM (2006) The reliability of isokinetic and isometric leg strength measures among individuals with symptoms of mild osteoarthritis. J Sports Med Phys Fitness 46:585–589
20. Hinman RS, Hunt MA, Creaby MW, Wrigley TV, McManus FJ, Bennell KL (2010) Hip muscle weakness in individuals with medial knee osteoarthritis. Arthritis Care Res 62(8):1190–1193
21. Marks R (1994) An investigation of the influence of age, clinical status, pain and position sense on stair walking in women with osteoarthrosis. Int J Rehabil Res 17:151–158
22. Sharma L (2003) Proprioception in osteoarthritis. In: Brandt KD, Doherty M, Lohmander LS (eds) Osteoarthritis, 2nd edn. Oxford Univ Press, Oxford, pp 172–177
23. Sharma L, Pai Y, Holtkamp K, Zev Rymer W (1997) Is knee proprioception worse in the arthritic knee versus the unaffected knee in unilateral knee osteoarthritis? Arthritis Rheum 40:1518–1525
24. Bennell KL, Hinman RS, Metcalf BR, Crossley KM, Buchbinder R, Smith M et al (2003) Relationship of knee joint proprioception to pain and disability in individuals with knee osteoarthritis. J Orthop Res 21:792–797
25. Marks R (1994) Correlation between knee position sense measurements and disease severity in persons with osteoarthritis. Rev Rheum Engl 61:365–372
26. Sharma L, Pai Y (1997) Impaired proprioception and osteoarthritis. Curr Opin Rheumatol 9:253–258
27. Sharma L (1999) Proprioceptive impairments in knee osteoarthritis. Rheu Dis Clin North Am 2:299–313
28. Garsden LR, Bullock-Saxton JE (1999) Joint reposition sense in subjects with unilateral osteoarthritis of the knee. Clin Rehabil 13:148–155
29. Sharma L (2004) The role of proprioceptive deficits, ligamentous laxity, and malalignment in development and progression of knee osteoarthritis. J Rheumatol 31(Suppl 70):87–92
30. Felson DT, Gross KD, Nevitt MC, Yang M, Lane NE, Torner JC, Lewis CE, Hurley MV (2009) The effects of impaired joint position sense on the development and progression of pain and structural damage in knee osteoarthritis. Arthritis Rheum 61(8):1070–1076
31. Hurkmans EJ, van der Esch M, Ostelo RW, Knol D, Dekker J, Steultjens MP (2007) Reproducibility of the measurement of knee joint proprioception in patients with osteoarthritis of the knee. Arthritis Rheum 57(8):1398–1403

32. Piriyaprasarth P, Morris ME, Winter A, Bialocerkowski AE (2008) The reliability of knee joint position testing using electrogoniometry. BMC Musculoskelet Disord 9:6
33. Segal NA, Glass NA, Felson DT, Hurley M, Yang M, Nevitt M, Lewis CE, Torner JC (2010) Effect of quadriceps strength and proprioception on risk for knee osteoarthritis. Med Sci Sports Exerc 42(11):2081–2088
34. Marks R, Quinney E, Wessel J (1993) Proprioceptive sensibility in women with normal and osteoarthritic knee joints. Clin Rheumatol 12:170–175
35. Thorlund JB, Shakoor N, Ageberg E, Sandal LF, Block JA, Roos EM (2012) Vibratory perception threshold in young and middle-aged patients at high risk of knee osteoarthritis compared to controls. Arthritis Care Res 64:144–148
36. Shakoor N, Lee KJ, Fogg LF, Wimmer MA, Foucher KC, Mikolaitis RA, Block JA (2012) The relationship of vibratory perception to dynamic joint loading, radiographic severity, and pain in knee osteoarthritis. Arthritis Rheum 64:181–186
37. Sharma L, Congron L, Felson DT, Dunlop DD, Kirwan-Mellis G, Hayes KW, Weinrach D, Buchanan T (1999) Laxity in healthy and osteoarthritic knees. Arthritis Rheum 42:861–870
38. Sharma L, Hayes KW, Felson DT, Buchanan TS, Kirwan-Mellis G, Lou C et al (1999) Does laxity alter the relationship between strength and physical function in knee osteoarthritis? Arthritis Rheum 42:25–32
39. Van der Esch M, Steultjens M, Ostelo RW, Harlaar J, Dekker J (2006) Reproducibility of instrumented knee joint laxity measurement in healthy subjects. Rheumatology (Oxford) 45:595–599
40. Van der Esch M, Steultjens M, Wieringa H, Dinant H, Dekker J (2005) Structural joint changes, malalignment, and laxity in osteoarthritis of the knee. Scand J Rheumatol 34:298–301
41. Yakhdani HR, Bafghi HA, Meijer OG, Bruijn SM, van den Dikkenberg N, Stibbe AB, van Royen BJ, van Dieen JH (2010) Stability and variability of knee kinematics during gait in knee osteoarthritis before and after replacement surgery. Clin Biomech 25:230–236
42. Bruijn SM, van Dieen JH, Meijer OG, Beek PJ (2009) Statistical precision and sensitivity of measures of dynamic gait stability. J Neurosci Methods 178:327–333
43. Felson DT, Niu J, McClennan C et al (2007) Knee buckling: prevalence, risk factors, and associated limitations in function. Ann Intern Med 147:534–540
44. Fitzgerald GK, Piva SR, Irrgang JJ (2004) Reports of joint instability in knee osteoarthritis: its prevalence and relationship to physical function. Arthritis Rheum 51:941–946
45. Knoop J, van der Leeden M, van der Esch M, Thorstensson C, Gerritsen M, Voorneman R, Lems WF, Roorda LD, Dekker J, Steultjens MPM (2012) Lower muscle strength is associated with self-reported knee instability in osteoarthritis of the knee: results from the AM-OA cohort. Arthritis Care Res 64:38–45
46. Fransen M, McConnell S, Hernandez-Molina G, Reichenbach S (2009) Exercise for osteoarthritis of the hip. Cochrane Database Syst Rev 3:CD007912
47. Van Baar ME, Dekker J, Oostendorp RA, Bijl D, Voorn TB, Lemmens JAM, Bijlsma JW (1998) The effectiveness of exercise therapy in patients with osteoarthritis of the hip or knee: a randomized clinical trial. Rheumatology 25:2432–2439
48. Steultjens MP, Dekker J, van Baar ME, Oostendorp RA, Bijlsma JW (2001) Muscle strength, pain and disability in patients with osteoarthritis. Clin Rehabil 15:331–341
49. Slemenda C, Brandt KD, Heilman DK, Mazzuca S, Braunstein EM, Katz BP et al (1997) Quadriceps weakness and osteoarthritis of the knee. Ann Intern Med 127:97–104
50. Thorstensson CA, Petersson IF, Jacobsson LT, Boegard TL, Roos EM (2004) Reduced functional performance in the lower extremity predicted radiographic knee osteoarthritis five years later. Ann Rheum Dis 63:402–407
51. Maly MR, Costigan PA, Olney SJ (2005) Contribution of psychosocial and mechanical variables to physical performance measures in knee osteoarthritis. Phys Ther 85:1318–1328

52. Holla JF, Steultjens MP, Roorda LD, Heymans MW, Ten Wolde S, Dekker J (2010) Prognostic factors for the two-year course of activity limitations in early osteoarthritis of the hip and/or knee. Arthritis Care Res (Hoboken) 62(10):1415–1425

53. van der Esch M, Steultjens M, Harlaar J, Wolterbeek N, Knol DL, Dekker J (2008) Knee varus-valgus motion during gait: a measure of joint stability in patients with osteoarthritis? Osteoarthritis Cartilage 16(4):522–525

54. Veenhof C, Huisman PA, Barten JA, Takken T, Pisters MF (2012) Factors associated with physical activity in patients with osteoarthritis of the hip or knee: a systematic review. Osteoarthritis Cartilage 20:6–12

Chapter 6
Behavioral Mechanisms Explaining Functional Decline

Jasmijn F.M. Holla, Martijn Pisters, and Joost Dekker

In Chap. 4, risk factors for functional decline in knee and hip OA patients are described. The chapter shows that: (1) the number of studies focusing on psychological, behavioral, and neuromuscular determinants of functional decline has increased considerably over the past 30 years; and (2) that pain, psychological distress (i.e., unpleasant mood states such as depression, anxiety, low vitality, and fatigue), pain coping behavior, low self-efficacy, and muscle weakness are associated with limitations in activity [1–10]. To be clinically useful, it should be known by means of which mechanisms these determinants cause limitations in activity in OA patients.

The avoidance model is a behavioral model that explains how behavioral mechanisms may lead to limitations in activity in knee OA patients. This chapter describes the avoidance model and reviews the current scientific evidence for the individual components of the model: pain during activity, psychological distress, avoidance of activity as a strategy to cope with pain, muscle weakness, and limitations in activity. Low self-efficacy [11–13] and pain-related fear [14–16] are also important determinants of limitations in activity in OA patients; however, these determinants are not included in the avoidance model. Therefore, the concepts of self-efficacy and pain-related fear will be described in a separate paragraph. Because the avoidance model is not fully applicable to hip OA, mechanisms in hip OA will also be discussed in a separate paragraph. At the end of the chapter, a summary is provided, and unresolved issues in need for further exploration are discussed.

J.F.M. Holla
Amsterdam Rehabilitation Research Center | Reade, Amsterdam, The Netherlands

M. Pisters
Clinical Health Sciences, University Medical Center Utrecht, Utrecht, The Netherlands

J. Dekker (✉)
Department of Rehabilitation Medicine, VU University Medical Center, PO Box 7057, 1007 MB Amsterdam, The Netherlands

Department of Psychiatry, VU University Medical Center, Amsterdam, The Netherlands
e-mail: j.dekker@vumc.nl

J. Dekker (ed.), *Exercise and Physical Functioning in Osteoarthritis: Medical, Neuromuscular and Behavioral Perspectives*, Springer Briefs in Specialty Topics in Behavioral Medicine, DOI 10.1007/978-1-4614-7215-5_6, © The Author(s) 2014

The Avoidance Model

Avoidance refers to behavior aimed at postponing or preventing an aversive situation from occurring [17]. If physical activity causes pain, avoidance of activity postpones or prevents pain [18]. At the short term, avoidance of activity reduces pain. However, the long-term effects of avoidance behavior can be negative, because physical inactivity is associated with more pain and more limitations in activity [5, 19].

During the past decades, several theoretical models have been developed to explain the associations between pain, avoidance, and limitations in activity in chronic pain patients [20]. The first models were based on the theories of classical and operant conditioning. In the models based on classical conditioning, it is assumed that pain becomes a conditioned stimulus for fear. The patient fears and avoids activities, which may cause pain; the patient becomes inactive, which leads to physical deconditioning and thereby limitations in activity [21, 22]. In the models based on operant conditioning, pain behaviors (e.g., avoidance, complaining, and use of analgesics) play an important role [21, 23]. It is assumed that these pain behaviors are reinforced and will therefore persist. For example, in the short term, avoidance of activity as reaction to acute pain may be reinforced by reduction of pain. In the longer term, avoidance of activity will lead to physical deconditioning and thereby limitations in activity. The latest models are based on the cognitive behavioral approach, based on the prevailing assumption that individuals actively process information regarding internal stimuli and external events [20]. These models emphasize the importance of cognitive processes in the development of chronic pain and limitations in activity [21, 24]. It is assumed that acute pain results in chronic pain in patients who use an adverse coping strategy such as catastrophizing [15, 21]. Dekker et al. [25] proposed a cognitive behavioral model to explain the development of limitations in activity in OA: the avoidance model. The avoidance model is based on operant and cognitive paradigms. Another well-known cognitive behavioral model of chronic pain is the fear-avoidance model [17, 26, 27]. This model has been developed in patients with low back pain, and will be described in section "Similarities and Differences with the Fear-Avoidance Model". The difference between the avoidance model and the fear-avoidance model will be described in section "Similarities and Differences with the Fear-Avoidance Model" as well.

The avoidance model [25, 28, 29] offers an explanation of how avoidance of activity leads to limitations in activity in patients with knee OA. According to this model (Fig. 6.1), a patient initially experiences pain during activity. This leads to the expectation that renewed activity results in more pain and consequently to avoidance of activity. In the short term, avoidance of activity may have the desired effect of less pain due to the decreased load on the affected joint. However, in the longer term, inactivity results in physical deconditioning, most notably muscle weakness. Muscle weakness leads to an increase in limitations in activity [29]. Psychological distress (e.g., anxiety, depression, low vitality, and fatigue) is associated with limitations in activity in OA [30, 31]. The avoidance model offers

Behavioral model

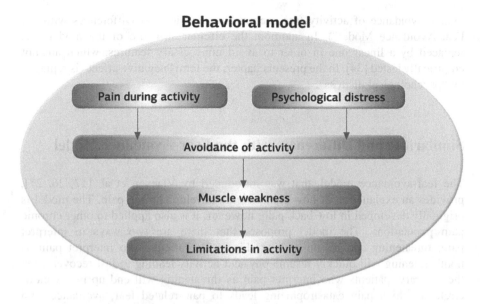

Fig. 6.1 The avoidance model

the following explanation for this phenomenon: it is hypothesized that psychological distress strengthens the tendency to avoid activity and thereby induces limitations in activity.

As shown in Fig. 6.1, the model hypothesizes an indirect relationship between pain during activity and muscle weakness via avoidance of activity. Avoidance of activity is hypothesized to mediate the relationship between pain and muscle weakness. A mediator variable is conceptualized as the mechanism through which one variable influences another variable [32, 33]. Likewise, the relationship between psychological distress and muscle weakness is hypothesized to be mediated by avoidance of activity, and the relationship between avoidance and limitations in activity is hypothesized to be mediated by muscle weakness.

The avoidance model underwent some development over the past years. The model that was published in 1993 included the constructs "pain," "negative affect," "low activity level," "muscle weakness," "instability of joints," and "disability" [28]. In the version of the model that was published in 2002, the term "low activity level" was replaced by the term "avoidance of activity," the construct "negative affect" was not used because negative affect was not evaluated in that study, and the construct "pain-related fear" was added [29]. In the latest version of the model that was published in 2012 [34], the terminology used was adapted to the International Classification of Functioning, Disability and Health (ICF) of the World Health Organization [35] (i.e., "limitations in activity" instead of "disability"). The construct "negative affect" was reintroduced, and the component "pain-related fear" was excluded based on the reasoning that the expectation of pain is sufficient to induce avoidance of activity (see section "Similarities and Differences with the Fear-Avoidance Model"). In addition, the circular structure of the model was replaced by a linear one in order to avoid unnecessary features, which are not empirically tested [34]. In the present chapter, the term "negative affect" is replaced by "psychological distress".

Similarities and Differences with the Fear-Avoidance Model

The fear-avoidance model, that was introduced by Vlaeyen et al. [17, 26, 27], provides an explanation of how pain patients develop chronic pain. The model is originally developed in low back pain; however, it is also applied to other chronic pain populations. The model proposes that there are two ways to interpret pain: threatening and nonthreatening (Fig. 6.2). Patients who interpret pain as nonthreatening will quickly resume physical activity leading to fast recovery. On the contrary, patients who interpret pain as threatening will end up in a vicious circle in which pain catastrophizing leads to pain-related fear, avoidance, and hypervigilance, with as consequence disuse, psychological distress, and limitations in activity [17, 26, 27].

Both the avoidance model and the fear-avoidance model describe the development of limitations in activity using the constructs pain, psychological distress, and avoidance. The most important differences between the avoidance model and the fear-avoidance model are (a) the absence of the term "pain-related fear" and (b) the inclusion of the neuromuscular component "muscle weakness" in the avoidance model.

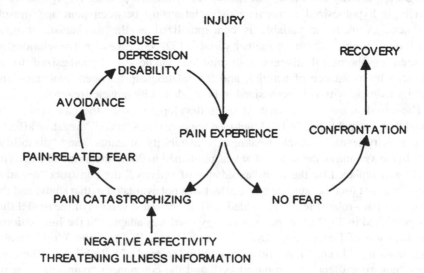

Fig. 6.2 The fear-avoidance model (*Source*: Vlaeyen JWS, Linton SJ. Fear-avoidance and its consequences in chronic musculoskeletal pain: a state of the art. Pain 2000;85:317–332 [27])

Pain-related fear was excluded from the avoidance model because it is hypothesized that avoidance behavior is not always caused by fear, it can also be caused by expectations. According to Bandura [36], outcome expectancy is defined as "a person's estimate that a given behavior will lead to certain outcomes" [36]. Efficacy expectancy is the "conviction that one can successfully execute the behavior required to produce the outcomes" [36]. Pain during activity is supposed to lead to avoidance of activity, because one has the outcome expectation that renewed activity will result in more pain. Efficacy expectations are so far not explicitly included in the avoidance model.

The neuromuscular component "muscle weakness" is explicitly included in the avoidance model and plays a central role. This distinguishes the avoidance model from other behavioral models in chronic pain. Whereas in the avoidance model the emphasis is on the mediating roles of avoidance and muscle weakness, in the fear-avoidance model the emphasis is on pain-related fear. Muscle weakness is also implicitly included in the fear-avoidance model under the term disuse; however, it has a much less central role [17].

The Components of the Avoidance Model

Below, we describe each of the components of the avoidance model and the instruments used to assess the components.

Pain

Pain, the unpleasant sensory and emotional experience associated with actual or potential tissue damage [37], is a main symptom of OA. It is a major reason for visits to the general practitioner in OA patients and is the most important cause of joint replacement surgery [38]. Initially, pain occurs after use of the affected joint during physical activity and is relieved by rest [28]. In later stages of OA, pain may also be present during rest [28, 39].

In OA, pain is usually measured with a visual analogue scale (VAS), a numeric rating scale (NRS) or a validated questionnaire. A VAS consists of a horizontal line, usually 100 mm in length, anchored by word descriptors at each end ("no pain" and "extreme pain"). The patient is asked to mark on the line the point that indicates pain intensity (at the present time, over the past week, etc.). The VAS score is determined by measuring in millimeters from the left end of the line to the point that the patient marks. An NRS consists of a horizontal set of numbers (0–10, 0–100, etc.), also anchored by word descriptors at each end. The patient is asked to mark the number that indicates pain intensity. Both the VAS and NRS have been shown to be reliable and valid measures of pain [40, 41]. Questionnaires that are widely used to measure pain in OA patients are the Western Ontario and McMaster Universities Osteoarthritis Index (WOMAC) [42] and the Short-Form 36 Health

Survey (SF-36) [43]. The WOMAC is a self-administered disease-specific questionnaire that assesses pain, stiffness, and limitations in activity in knee and hip OA using a battery of 24 questions [42]. The WOMAC is available in a 5-point Likert, 100-mm VAS, and 11-box NRS format and has been shown to be reliable, valid, and responsive [42, 44]. Two of the five items of the pain subscale of the WOMAC concern pain during activity (i.e., "How much pain have you had when walking on a flat surface?" and "How much pain have you had when going up or down stairs?"). The SF-36 is a generic questionnaire that assesses health-related quality of life [43]. The questionnaire has been shown to be reliable, valid, and responsive in different patient groups including OA [43, 44]. The pain subscale of the SF-36 consists of two items that are answered on a 5-point Likert scale [i.e., "How much bodily pain have you had during the past 4 weeks?" and "During the past 4 weeks, how much did pain interfere with your normal work (including both work outside the home and housework)?"].

Psychological Distress

Psychological distress refers to a broad range of unpleasant mood states such as depression, anxiety, low vitality, and fatigue. A depressed and anxious mood is more prevalent in OA patients than in healthy persons [45, 46]. Likewise, fatigue is common in OA [47]. Psychological distress has frequently been associated with limitations in activity in OA patients [30, 34, 48–51]. Social withdrawal and isolation are important consequences of psychological distress [52, 53]. In the avoidance model, psychological distress is hypothesized to strengthen the tendency to avoid activity.

Psychological distress is usually measured using self-administered questionnaires. Questionnaires that are often used to measure psychological distress in OA patients are: the Hospital Anxiety and Depression Scale (HADS) [54], the Symptom Checklist-90 (SCL-90) [55] (i.e., a generic instrument that helps to evaluate a broad range of psychological problems and symptoms of psychopathology), the Center for the Epidemiologic Studies Depression scale (CES-D) [56], and the SF-36 [43] subscale for mental health. Fatigue is often measured using a VAS or NRS. The opposite of fatigue, i.e., vitality, is frequently assessed with the vitality subscale of the SF-36 [43].

Avoidance of Activity

Avoidance refers to behavior aimed at deferring or preventing an aversive situation from occurring [17]. If physical activity causes pain, one will tend to avoid activity to prevent pain from occurring [18]. For example, if stair-climbing causes pain, one will tend to take the elevator.

Avoidance of activity is commonly studied under the category "pain coping," defined as behavioral and cognitive attempts to manage or tolerate pain and its effects [57]. Pain coping can be classified into active strategies such as relieving, controlling, or functioning with pain, and passive strategies that include negative self-statements about pain, catastrophizing (i.e., the tendency to focus on and exaggerate the threat value of painful stimuli and negatively evaluate one's ability to deal with pain) [58], withdrawal, and avoidance of activity [57]. In the avoidance model, the passive pain coping strategy "avoidance of activity" plays a key role; it starts the process of physical deconditioning, which subsequently leads to limitations in activity.

In most studies on avoidance behavior in OA patients, avoidance of activity is measured using self-report questionnaires. So far, all studies aimed at validating the avoidance model used the resting subscale of the Pain Coping Inventory [57] as measure of avoidance of activity [29, 34, 59]. Physical activity is often measured with the Physical Activity Scale for the Elderly (PASE): a brief self-report instrument for the assessment of leisure-time, household, and work-related physical activity in older people [60]. However, it is generally agreed that assessment of avoidance should strive to cover subjective and objective aspects of avoidance behavior [27]. Thus, while self-report questionnaires are important, recordings are also valuable in measuring avoidance of activity [27, 34]. An accelerometer can be used to measure objective levels of physical activity [61]. The accelerometer is a small device that is worn by the patient for a certain period. The device detects accelerations, which are converted into activity counts per minute, indicating the level of activity.

Muscle Weakness

Muscle weakness is a reduction in the strength of one or more muscles. Several studies have demonstrated that quadriceps weakness occurs early in OA and is an important determinant of limitations in activity [2, 6, 62, 63]. Enduring avoidance of activity may result in physical deconditioning, which can be expressed in muscle weakness, reduced aerobic fitness, and disordered muscle coordination [17]. Muscle weakness is included in the avoidance model as measure of physical deconditioning. It is hypothesized that muscle weakness mediates the association between avoidance and limitations in activity.

The assessment of muscle weakness involves the measurement of muscle strength of several muscle actions of different joints [6]. The large amount of data resulting from these measurements is usually reduced into one or more sum scores. Often muscle strength around the most affected knee or hip, or the average muscle strength of the right and left leg, is used in the analyses. More information on these sum scores and the measurement methods of muscle weakness used in OA patients is given in Chap. 5. In studies that examined the mediating role of muscle strength in patients with knee OA, the average strength of the knee extensors (quadriceps) and knee flexors (hamstrings) of the most affected leg is mostly used as measure of muscle weakness [29, 34, 59]. One study examined the mediating role of muscle strength in patients with knee or hip OA. In this study, the average muscle strength of the knee extensors and hip abductors was used as measure of muscle weakness in the analyses [59].

Limitations in Activity

Limitations in activity are defined as difficulties an individual may have in executing activities in the ICF [35]. Limitations in activity are usually assessed with self-report questionnaires (e.g., the physical function subscales of the WOMAC and SF-36) and performance-based tests such as a 100-m walk test or a stair climbing test.

More information on these measurement methods is already given in Chap. 5. The avoidance model hypothesizes that prolonged avoidance behavior leads to muscle weakness and thereby limitations in activity.

Related Constructs

Several studies have shown that besides pain, psychological distress, and avoidance of activity, the concepts of self-efficacy [11–13] and pain-related fear [14–16] might be relevant to explain limitations in activity in OA patients. These concepts are not included in the avoidance model. Therefore, these constructs will be shortly described here.

Self-Efficacy. Self-efficacy is part of the social cognitive theory that was founded by Bandura [36]. According to this theory, the human behavior is greatly determined by one's expectations regarding specific behavior. A distinction is made between outcome expectations (i.e., one's estimate that a given behavior causes a certain outcome) and efficacy expectations or self-efficacy. Self-efficacy is defined as the conviction that one can successfully execute the behavior required to complete a task or activity [12, 36]. Outcome expectations differ from efficacy expectations, when a person expects that a particular activity will lead to a certain outcome but is unsure that he/she is able to perform this activity. The level of self-efficacy determines to what degree a person will devote his/her energy to accomplish a task; it affects both the initiation and the persistence of coping behavior [36]. In OA patients, self-efficacy is mostly measured with the Arthritis Self-Efficacy Scale (ASES) [64]. The ASES is a disease-specific self-report questionnaire consisting of 20 items that assess the patient's belief that he/she can complete tasks related to physical function and pain or symptom management. The questionnaire consists of three subscales: physical function, pain, and other symptoms. The patients have to rate how certain they are of their ability to complete a task or control pain or other symptoms on a 100-mm VAS or NRS [64].

Pain-Related Fear. Pain-related fear, defined as the fear that emerges when stimuli that are related to pain are perceived as a main threat, plays a central role in the fear-avoidance model [17, 27]. It is suggested that pain-related fear contributes to interindividual variations in pain in OA patients [15]. In OA patients, pain-related fear is mostly measured with the Tampa Scale for Kinesiophobia (TSK) [65]: a 17-item self-report questionnaire that is aimed at the assessment of fear of (re)injury due to movement [14].

Scientific Evidence for the Avoidance Model

Several studies have demonstrated direct associations between pain [3, 9, 34, 66, 67], psychological distress [34, 66, 68], avoidance of activity [5, 10, 29, 34, 69], muscle weakness [6, 9, 29, 34], and limitations in activity in knee OA patients. These studies provide some support for the avoidance model. Stronger evidence has been obtained in studies testing mediation and prognostic studies. Since the introduction of the avoidance model in OA patients in 1992 [25], four such studies were done [28, 29, 34, 59]. Besides these studies purposefully aiming at validation of the avoidance model, several studies evaluated interrelationships between components of the model, without explicitly testing the avoidance model. These studies are summarized below.

Pain—Avoidance of Activity—Muscle Weakness

In the avoidance model, it is hypothesized that pain during activity leads to muscle weakness via avoidance of activity (mediation of avoidance, see Fig. 6.1). In a recent study, we verified and confirmed the validity of this hypothesis in patients with early symptomatic knee OA [34]. In this cross-sectional study, among 151 patients we found that pain during activity was positively associated with avoidance of activity, indicating that patients who reported higher levels of pain were more inclined to avoid physical activity [34]. Avoidance of activity was found to be negatively associated with muscle strength around the knee, indicating that patients who reported higher levels of avoidance had weaker muscles. Pain was found to be negatively associated with muscle strength, both directly and indirectly. This finding indicates that patients who reported higher levels of pain had weaker muscles, because these patients were more inclined to avoid activity. Because the study was aimed at validating the whole avoidance model, the associations between pain, avoidance, and muscle strength were examined in one structural equation model together with psychological distress and limitations in activity (see Fig. 6.1).

Psychological Distress—Avoidance of Activity—Muscle Weakness

In the same study [34], psychological distress was measured with the subscales for mental health and vitality of the SF-36 [43]. We found that avoidance of activity indeed mediated the association between psychological distress and muscle strength.

Avoidance of Activity—Limitations in Activity

Steultjens et al. [5] examined the role of coping styles as predictors for pain and limitations in activity 36 weeks later in 119 patients with knee OA. Avoidance of activity was found to predict a higher degree of limitations in activity 36 weeks later. Similarly, Pisters et al. [10] found that avoidance of activity was an important predictor for limitations in activity over 5 years in 216 patients with knee OA. Perrot et al. [70] reported a cross-sectional association between avoidance and limitations in activity in 2,781 patients with knee OA. They also reported that OA patients more frequently avoided activity than patients with rheumatoid arthritis [70]. These authors suggested that in OA patients, pain is increased by physical activity, whereas in RA patients, pain mostly occurs in the morning and is usually relieved by physical activity [70]. Several other studies have shown that OA patients who use passive coping strategies such as catastrophizing, helplessness, and avoidance of activity, report higher levels of pain and more limitations in activity [4, 7, 15, 16, 71–77].

Avoidance of Activity—Muscle Weakness—Limitations in Activity

Two cross-sectional studies examined the hypothesis that muscle weakness plays a mediating role in the relationship between avoidance and limitations in activity in knee OA patients [29, 34]. The first study was conducted in 107 patients with clinical knee OA and a mean age of 69 years [29]. The second study was conducted in 151 patients with early symptomatic knee OA with a mean age of 59 years [34]. Both studies confirmed that avoidance leads to limitations in activity via muscle weakness. The results of the second study support the assumption that the relationships described in the avoidance model are initiated early in the disease process, because in this stage patients experience activity-related pain for the first time, leading to the described process of adaptation.

A limitation of both mentioned studies is that a cross-sectional design was used to study a model describing longitudinal relationships. As a result, no causalities can be implied. One study so far examined the mediating role of muscle weakness using a longitudinal design [59]. The study population of this study consisted of 216 patients with knee OA with a mean age of 66 years old. Measurements were conducted at baseline, and after 1, 2, 3, and 5 years of follow-up. The data were analyzed using generalized estimating equations (GEE) analyses. Avoidance of activity was found to be negatively associated with muscle strength and to be positively associated with limitations in activity. Muscle strength was found to be negatively associated with limitations in activity. In an analysis with avoidance of activity and muscle strength as independent variables and limitations in activity as dependent variable, the impact of avoidance on limitations in activity was reduced compared with an analysis with only avoidance of activity as independent variable. These results confirm the mediating role of muscle strength in the association between avoidance and limitations in activity.

All three studies examining the mediating role of muscle strength in the avoidance model found that avoidance of activity was both directly and indirectly associated with limitations in activity [29, 34]. This indicates that the association between avoidance and limitations in activity is partly mediated by muscle weakness. Apparently, there are also other pathways via which avoidance of activity has an influence on limitations in activity.

Other Behavioral Mechanisms

Resilience—Self-Efficacy—Pain and Limitations in Activity

Wright et al. [78] examined the association between psychological distress, resilience (i.e., vitality, positive effect, and extraversion), self-efficacy, pain, and limitations in activity in 275 patients with early knee OA. They found that patients who reported higher levels of self-efficacy reported less pain and limitations in activity. In addition, they found that the effect of resilience on pain was mediated by self-efficacy: greater resilience was associated with less pain and limitations in activity via a higher level of self-efficacy [78]. Two other studies reported associations between self-efficacy and pain [11] and limitations in activity [11, 12]. Finally, an association between self-efficacy and psychological distress has been shown; Maly et al. [79] reported a negative association between depressed mood and self-efficacy.

Pain—Pain-Related Fear—Limitations in Activity

Heuts et al. [14] examined the associations between pain intensity, pain-related fear, and limitations in activity in a sample of 254 patients with knee and/or hip OA. They found that both pain intensity and pain-related fear were positively associated with limitations in activity. Two other studies examined the association between pain-related fear and limitations in activity in knee OA patients and found comparable results [15, 16]. Somers et al. [15] found that pain-related fear explained a significant proportion of the variance in walking at a fast speed in 106 patients with knee OA. Sullivan et al. [16] found that pain-related fear was associated with limitations in activity after total knee arthroplasty. However, after adjustment for presurgical comorbidities, this association was no longer significant.

Hip Osteoarthritis

Muscle weakness as the explanation of the association between avoidance and limitations in activity is not (fully) applicable to hip OA patients. Whereas the knee joint is particularly stabilized by muscle strength, the stability of the hip joint is to a large extent provided by its shape (i.e., ball and socket joint). Therefore, it is hypothesized that muscle weakness plays a less important role in the development of limitations in activity in hip OA patients than in knee OA patients. This hypothesis was confirmed in a recent study in which the mediating role of muscle strength in the association between avoidance and limitations in activity was assessed in both patients with hip OA ($n = 149$) and patients with knee OA ($n = 216$). The mean age of the study population was 66 years old. Measurements were conducted at baseline, and after 1, 2, 3, and 5 years of follow-up, and the data were analyzed using generalized estimating equations (GEE) analyses. In this longitudinal study, the mediating role of muscle strength was confirmed in patients with knee OA but not in patients with hip OA [59].

On the other hand, Pisters et al. [10] found that avoidance of activity is an important predictor for limitations in activity in both hip and knee OA. Hawker et al. [38] found that both hip and knee OA patients who experience intense, unpredictable pain that affects their mood tend to avoid social and recreational activities. Also, Rosemann et al. [80] found that more pain is associated with a lower level of physical activity in hip OA patients. Finally, associations between depressed mood [81, 82] and fatigue [83] and a lower level of physical activity in hip OA patients are reported. Therefore, also in hip OA, there is evidence that avoidance of activity plays a role. However, the mechanism via which avoidance contributes to the development of limitations in activity in hip OA patients is not clear. Contrary to in knee OA, it is less likely that muscle weakness plays a mediating role. Further research is needed to explain the role of avoidance of activity in hip OA.

Conclusion and Unexplored Issues

The avoidance model is a behavioral model that explains how behavioral mechanisms may lead to limitations in activity in knee OA patients. This chapter described the avoidance model and reviewed the current scientific evidence for the individual components of the model: pain during activity, psychological distress, avoidance of activity as a coping strategy, muscle weakness, and limitations in activity. In addition, the associations between self-efficacy and pain-related fear and limitations in activity were described.

It can be concluded that the results of the studies so far provide evidence for the validity of the avoidance model as described in Fig. 6.1. Most evidence is obtained from cross-sectional studies. There is a need for longitudinal studies to test the causal relationships as described in the model. Furthermore, the indirect association between pain and limitations in activity via avoidance and muscle weakness accounts for a part of the total association between pain and limitations in activity [29, 34]. This indicates that there are other pathways between pain and limitations in activity than those hypothesized in the avoidance model. Alternative pathways may involve poor voluntary effort [84] or low self-efficacy beliefs [29]. Likewise, the indirect association between psychological distress and limitations in activity accounts for part of the total association between psychological distress and limitations in activity [34]. Again, this finding indicates that avoidance is not the only mechanism explaining limitations in activity in knee and hip OA: avoidance is one mechanism, among other mechanisms.

Because risk factors for functional decline differ between knee and hip OA patients, it is likely that also the underlying mechanisms differ. Most studies examining behavioral mechanisms leading to the development of limitations in activity in OA focus on knee OA. As a result, in hip OA, less is known about these mechanisms. Therefore, more research is needed in hip OA.

Knowledge of mechanisms leading to limitations in activity in OA patients is important for improvement of targeted exercise interventions. For patients with avoidance behavior, an intervention aimed at an increase in daily physical activity using a cognitive-behavioral approach seems suitable [85]. This kind of interventions will be described in Chap. 9.

References

1. Botha-Scheepers S, Riyazi N, Kroon HM, Scharloo M, Houwing-Duistermaat JJ, Slagboom E et al (2006) Activity limitations in the lower extremities in patients with osteoarthritis: the modifying effects of illness perceptions and mental health. Osteoarthritis Cartilage 14 (11):1104–1110
2. Dekker J, van Dijk GM, Veenhof C (2009) Risk factors for functional decline in osteoarthritis of the hip or knee. Curr Opin Rheumatol 21(5):520–524
3. Holla JF, Steultjens MP, Roorda LD, Heymans MW, Ten Wolde S, Dekker J (2010) Prognostic factors for the two-year course of activity limitations in early osteoarthritis of the hip and/or knee. Arthritis Care Res (Hoboken) 62(10):1415–1425
4. Hopman-Rock M, Kraaimaat FW, Odding E, Bijlsma JW (1998) Coping with pain in the hip or knee in relation to physical disability in community-living elderly people. Arthritis Care Res 11(4):243–252
5. Steultjens MP, Dekker J, Bijlsma JW (2001) Coping, pain, and disability in osteoarthritis: a longitudinal study. J Rheumatol 28(5):1068–1072
6. Steultjens MP, Dekker J, van Baar ME, Oostendorp RA, Bijlsma JW (2001) Muscle strength, pain and disability in patients with osteoarthritis. Clin Rehabil 15(3):331–341

 7. van Baar ME, Dekker J, Lemmens JA, Oostendorp RA, Bijlsma JW (1998) Pain and disability in patients with osteoarthritis of hip or knee: the relationship with articular, kinesiological, and psychological characteristics. J Rheumatol 25(1):125–133
 8. van Dijk GM, Dekker J, Veenhof C, van den Ende CH (2006) Course of functional status and pain in osteoarthritis of the hip or knee: a systematic review of the literature. Arthritis Rheum 55(5):779–785
 9. van Dijk GM, Veenhof C, Spreeuwenberg P, Coene N, Burger BJ, van Schaardenburg D et al (2010) Prognosis of limitations in activities in osteoarthritis of the hip or knee: a three year cohort study. Arch Phys Med Rehabil 91(1):58–66
10. Pisters MF, Veenhof C, van Dijk GM, Heymans MW, Twisk JW, Dekker J (2012) The course of limitations in activities over 5 years in patients with knee and hip osteoarthritis with moderate functional limitations: risk factors for future functional decline. Osteoarthritis Cartilage 20(6):503–510
11. Pells JJ, Shelby RA, Keefe FJ, Dixon KE, Blumenthal JA, Lacaille L et al (2008) Arthritis self-efficacy and self-efficacy for resisting eating: relationships to pain, disability, and eating behavior in overweight and obese individuals with osteoarthritic knee pain. Pain 136 (3):340–347
12. Harrison AL (2004) The influence of pathology, pain, balance, and self-efficacy on function in women with osteoarthritis of the knee. Phys Ther 84(9):822–831
13. Rejeski WJ, Craven T, Ettinger WH Jr, McFarlane M, Shumaker S (1996) Self-efficacy and pain in disability with osteoarthritis of the knee. J Gerontol B Psychol Sci Soc Sci 51(1):24–29
14. Heuts PH, Vlaeyen JW, Roelofs J, de Bie RA, Aretz K, van Weel C et al (2004) Pain-related fear and daily functioning in patients with osteoarthritis. Pain 110(1–2):228–235
15. Somers TJ, Keefe FJ, Pells JJ, Dixon KE, Waters SJ, Riordan PA et al (2009) Pain catastrophizing and pain-related fear in osteoarthritis patients: relationships to pain and disability. J Pain Symptom Manage 37(5):863–872
16. Sullivan M, Tanzer M, Stanish W, Fallaha M, Keefe FJ, Simmonds M et al (2009) Psychological determinants of problematic outcomes following Total Knee Arthroplasty. Pain 143 (1–2):123–129
17. Leeuw M, Goossens ME, Linton SJ, Crombez G, Boersma K, Vlaeyen JW (2007) The fear-avoidance model of musculoskeletal pain: current state of scientific evidence. J Behav Med 30(1):77–94
18. Philips HC (1987) Avoidance behaviour and its role in sustaining chronic pain. Behav Res Ther 25(4):273–279
19. Kaplan MS, Huguet N, Newsom JT, McFarland BH (2003) Characteristics of physically inactive older adults with arthritis: results of a population-based study. Prev Med 37(1):61–67
20. Linton SJ (2002) New avenues for the prevention of chronic musculoskeletal pain and disability. Elsevier Health Sciences, Amsterdam
21. Turk DC, Flor H (1984) Etiological theories and treatments for chronic back pain. II. Psychological models and interventions. Pain 19(3):209–233
22. Gentry WD, Bernal GAA (1977) Chronic pain. In: Williams RB, Gentry WD (eds) Behavioral approaches to medical treatment. Ballinger, Cambridge, MA, pp 173–182
23. Fordyce WE (1978) Learning processes in pain. In: Sternbach RA (ed) The psychology of pain. Raven, New York, pp 5–42
24. Meichenbaum DH, Turk DC (1976) The cognitive management of anxiety, depression and pain. In: Davidson PO (ed) The behavioral management of anxiety, depression and pain. Brunner/Mazel, New York, pp 1–34
25. Dekker J, Boot B, van der Woude LH, Bijlsma JW (1992) Pain and disability in osteoarthritis: a review of biobehavioral mechanisms. J Behav Med 15(2):189–214
26. Vlaeyen JW, Kole-Snijders AM, Boeren RG, van Eek H (1995) Fear of movement/(re)injury in chronic low back pain and its relation to behavioral performance. Pain 62(3):363–372
27. Vlaeyen JW, Linton SJ (2000) Fear-avoidance and its consequences in chronic musculoskeletal pain: a state of the art. Pain 85(3):317–332

28. Dekker J, Tola P, Aufdemkampe G, Winckers M (1993) Negative affect, pain and disability in osteoarthritis patients: the mediating role of muscle weakness. Behav Res Ther 31(2):203–206
29. Steultjens MP, Dekker J, Bijlsma JW (2002) Avoidance of activity and disability in patients with osteoarthritis of the knee: the mediating role of muscle strength. Arthritis Rheum 46(7):1784–1788
30. Somers TJ, Keefe FJ, Godiwala N, Hoyler GH (2009) Psychosocial factors and the pain experience of osteoarthritis patients: new findings and new directions. Curr Opin Rheumatol 21(5):501–506
31. Knoop J, van der Leeden M, Thorstensson CA, Roorda LD, Lems WF, Knol DL et al (2011) Identification of phenotypes with different clinical outcomes in knee osteoarthritis: data from the Osteoarthritis Initiative. Arthritis Care Res (Hoboken) 63(11):1535–1542
32. Baron RM, Kenny DA (1986) The moderator-mediator variable distinction in social psychological research: conceptual, strategic, and statistical considerations. J Pers Soc Psychol 51(6):1173–1182
33. Rose BM, Holmbeck GN, Coakley RM, Franks EA (2004) Mediator and moderator effects in developmental and behavioral pediatric research. J Dev Behav Pediatr 25(1):58–67
34. Holla JF, van der Leeden M, Knol DL, Peter WF, Roorda LD, Lems WF et al (2012) Avoidance of activities in early symptomatic knee osteoarthritis: results from the CHECK cohort. Ann Behav Med 44(1):33–42
35. World Health Organization (2001) International classification of functioning, disability and health: ICF. WHO, Geneva
36. Bandura A (1977) Self-efficacy: toward a unifying theory of behavioral change. Psychol Rev 84(2):191–215
37. International Association for the Study of Pain Task Force on Taxonomy (1994) Classification of chronic pain: description of chronic pain syndromes and definition of pain terms, 2nd edn. IASP Press, Seattle
38. Hawker GA, Stewart L, French MR, Cibere J, Jordan JM, March L et al (2008) Understanding the pain experience in hip and knee osteoarthritis–an OARSI/OMERACT initiative. Osteoarthritis Cartilage 16(4):415–422
39. Woolhead G, Gooberman-Hill R, Dieppe P, Hawker G (2010) Night pain in hip and knee osteoarthritis: a focus group study. Arthritis Care Res (Hoboken) 62(7):944–949
40. Williamson A, Hoggart B (2005) Pain: a review of three commonly used pain rating scales. J Clin Nurs 14(7):798–804
41. Langley GB, Sheppeard H (1985) The visual analogue scale: its use in pain measurement. Rheumatol Int 5(4):145–148
42. Bellamy N, Buchanan WW, Goldsmith CH, Campbell J, Stitt LW (1988) Validation study of WOMAC: a health status instrument for measuring clinically important patient relevant outcomes to antirheumatic drug therapy in patients with osteoarthritis of the hip or knee. J Rheumatol 15(12):1833–1840
43. Ware JE Jr, Sherbourne CD (1992) The MOS 36-item short-form health survey (SF-36). I. Conceptual framework and item selection. Med Care 30(6):473–483
44. Veenhof C, Bijlsma JW, van den Ende CH, van Dijk GM, Pisters MF, Dekker J (2006) Psychometric evaluation of osteoarthritis questionnaires: a systematic review of the literature. Arthritis Rheum 55(3):480–492
45. Axford J, Butt A, Heron C, Hammond J, Morgan J, Alavi A et al (2010) Prevalence of anxiety and depression in osteoarthritis: use of the Hospital Anxiety and Depression Scale as a screening tool. Clin Rheumatol 29(11):1277–1283
46. Lin EH (2008) Depression and osteoarthritis. Am J Med 121(11 Suppl 2):S16–S19
47. Wolfe F, Hawley DJ, Wilson K (1996) The prevalence and meaning of fatigue in rheumatic disease. J Rheumatol 23(8):1407–1417
48. Scopaz KA, Piva SR, Wisniewski S, Fitzgerald GK (2009) Relationships of fear, anxiety, and depression with physical function in patients with knee osteoarthritis. Arch Phys Med Rehabil 90(11):1866–1873

49. O'Reilly SC, Muir KR, Doherty M (1998) Knee pain and disability in the Nottingham community: association with poor health status and psychological distress. Br J Rheumatol 37(8):870–873
50. Murphy SL, Smith DM (2010) Ecological measurement of fatigue and fatigability in older adults with osteoarthritis. J Gerontol A Biol Sci Med Sci 65(2):184–189
51. Parmelee PA, Harralson TL, Smith LA, Schumacher HR (2007) Necessary and discretionary activities in knee osteoarthritis: do they mediate the pain-depression relationship? Pain Med 8(5):449–461
52. American Psychiatric Association (1994) Diagnostic and statistical manual of mental disorders, 4th edn. Author, Washington, DC
53. Ridner SH (2004) Psychological distress: concept analysis. J Adv Nurs 45(5):536–545
54. Zigmond AS, Snaith RP (1983) The hospital anxiety and depression scale. Acta Psychiatr Scand 67(6):361–370
55. Derogatis LR, Lipman RS, Covi L (1973) SCL-90: an outpatient psychiatric rating scale–preliminary report. Psychopharmacol Bull 9(1):13–28
56. Radloff LS (1977) The CES-D scale: a self-report depression scale for research in the general population. Appl Psychol Meas 1:385–401
57. Kraaimaat FW, Evers AW (2003) Pain-coping strategies in chronic pain patients: psychometric characteristics of the pain-coping inventory (PCI). Int J Behav Med 10(4):343–363
58. Keefe FJ, Lefebvre JC, Egert JR, Affleck G, Sullivan MJ, Caldwell DS (2000) The relationship of gender to pain, pain behavior, and disability in osteoarthritis patients: the role of catastrophizing. Pain 87(3):325–334
59. Pisters MF, Veenhof C, van Dijk GM, Dekker J (submitted for publication) Avoidance of activity and limitations in activities in patients with osteoarthritis of the hip or knee: a five year follow up study on the mediating role of reduced muscle strength
60. Washburn RA, Smith KW, Jette AM, Janney CA (1993) The Physical Activity Scale for the Elderly (PASE): development and evaluation. J Clin Epidemiol 46(2):153–162
61. Bassett DR Jr, Ainsworth BE, Swartz AM, Strath SJ, O'Brien WL, King GA (2000) Validity of four motion sensors in measuring moderate intensity physical activity. Med Sci Sports Exerc 32(9 Suppl):S471–S480
62. Roos EM, Herzog W, Block JA, Bennell KL (2011) Muscle weakness, afferent sensory dysfunction and exercise in knee osteoarthritis. Nat Rev Rheumatol 7(1):57–63
63. Hurley MV (2003) Muscle dysfunction and effective rehabilitation of knee osteoarthritis: what we know and what we need to find out. Arthritis Rheum 49(3):444–452
64. Lorig K, Chastain RL, Ung E, Shoor S, Holman HR (1989) Development and evaluation of a scale to measure perceived self-efficacy in people with arthritis. Arthritis Rheum 32(1):37–44
65. Kori S, Miller R, Todd D (1990) Kinesiophobia: a new view of chronic pain behavior. Pain Manage 3:35–43
66. Mallen CD, Peat G, Thomas E, Lacey R, Croft P (2007) Predicting poor functional outcome in community-dwelling older adults with knee pain: prognostic value of generic indicators. Ann Rheum Dis 66(11):1456–1461
67. Thomas E, Peat G, Mallen C, Wood L, Lacey R, Duncan R et al (2008) Predicting the course of functional limitation among older adults with knee pain: do local signs, symptoms and radiographs add anything to general indicators? Ann Rheum Dis 67(10):1390–1398
68. Riddle DL, Kong X, Fitzgerald GK (2011) Psychological health impact on 2-year changes in pain and function in persons with knee pain: data from the Osteoarthritis Initiative. Osteoarthritis Cartilage 19(9):1095–1101
69. Dunlop DD, Semanik P, Song J, Manheim LM, Shih V, Chang RW (2005) Risk factors for functional decline in older adults with arthritis. Arthritis Rheum 52(4):1274–1282
70. Perrot S, Poiraudeau S, Kabir M, Bertin P, Sichere P, Serrie A et al (2008) Active or passive pain coping strategies in hip and knee osteoarthritis? Results of a national survey of 4,719 patients in a primary care setting. Arthritis Rheum 59(11):1555–1562

71. Shelby RA, Somers TJ, Keefe FJ, Pells JJ, Dixon KE, Blumenthal JA (2008) Domain specific self-efficacy mediates the impact of pain catastrophizing on pain and disability in overweight and obese osteoarthritis patients. J Pain 9(10):912–919
72. Rapp SR, Rejeski WJ, Miller ME (2000) Physical function among older adults with knee pain: the role of pain coping skills. Arthritis Care Res 13(5):270–279
73. Keefe FJ, Caldwell DS, Queen K, Gil KM, Martinez S, Crisson JE et al (1987) Osteoarthritic knee pain: a behavioral analysis. Pain 28(3):309–321
74. France CR, Keefe FJ, Emery CF, Affleck G, France JL, Waters S et al (2004) Laboratory pain perception and clinical pain in post-menopausal women and age-matched men with osteoarthritis: relationship to pain coping and hormonal status. Pain 112(3):274–281
75. Edwards RR, Bingham CO III, Bathon J, Haythornthwaite JA (2006) Catastrophizing and pain in arthritis, fibromyalgia, and other rheumatic diseases. Arthritis Rheum 55(2):325–332
76. Creamer P, Lethbridge-Cejku M, Hochberg MC (1999) Determinants of pain severity in knee osteoarthritis: effect of demographic and psychosocial variables using 3 pain measures. J Rheumatol 26(8):1785–1792
77. Creamer P, Lethbridge-Cejku M, Hochberg MC (2000) Factors associated with functional impairment in symptomatic knee osteoarthritis. Rheumatology (Oxford) 39(5):490–496
78. Wright LJ, Zautra AJ, Going S (2008) Adaptation to early knee osteoarthritis: the role of risk, resilience, and disease severity on pain and physical functioning. Ann Behav Med 36(1):70–80
79. Maly MR, Costigan PA, Olney SJ (2006) Determinants of self efficacy for physical tasks in people with knee osteoarthritis. Arthritis Rheum 55(1):94–101
80. Rosemann T, Laux G, Szecsenyi J, Wensing M, Grol R (2008) Pain and osteoarthritis in primary care: factors associated with pain perception in a sample of 1,021 patients. Pain Med 9(7):903–910
81. Veenhof C, Huisman PA, Barten JA, Takken T, Pisters MF (2012) Factors associated with physical activity in patients with osteoarthritis of the hip or knee: a systematic review. Osteoarthritis Cartilage 20(1):6–12
82. de Groot IB, Bussmann JB, Stam HJ, Verhaar JA (2008) Actual everyday physical activity in patients with end-stage hip or knee osteoarthritis compared with healthy controls. Osteoarthritis Cartilage 16(4):436–442
83. Murphy SL, Smith DM, Clauw DJ, Alexander NB (2008) The impact of momentary pain and fatigue on physical activity in women with osteoarthritis. Arthritis Rheum 59(6):849–856
84. O'Reilly SC, Jones A, Muir KR, Doherty M (1998) Quadriceps weakness in knee osteoarthritis: the effect on pain and disability. Ann Rheum Dis 57(10):588–594
85. Veenhof C, van den Ende CH, Dekker J, Kiike AJ, Oostendorp RA, Bijlsma JW (2007) Which patients with osteoarthritis of hip and/or knee benefit most from behavioral graded activity? Int J Behav Med 14(2):86–91

Part III
Exercise Therapy

Chapter 7
Regular Exercises in Knee and Hip Osteoarthritis

Marike van der Leeden, Wilfred Peter, and Joost Dekker

Exercise consists of planned, structured, and repetitive bodily movement designed to improve or maintain one or more components of physical fitness [1]. Performing exercises and being physically active are key recommendations in current guidelines for the management of osteoarthritis (OA) of the knee and hip [2–8]. In knee OA, exercises have been found to relieve pain and to reduce activity limitations [9–11], with small-to-moderate effect sizes. In hip OA, exercises are likely to be effective, although limited evidence is available [12].

The present chapter provides information on regular exercises in knee and hip OA, based on evidence from the literature. Regular exercises include exercises aiming at improvement of muscle strength, aerobic capacity, flexibility, and daily activities. Exercises can be performed under supervision (individually or in a group) or unsupervised at home.

Muscle Strengthening Exercises

Muscle weakness is a common feature of knee and hip OA and has been found to be strongly associated with limitations in daily activities [13, 14]. Likewise, muscle strengthening exercises are regarded the most important component of exercise therapy in patients with knee and hip OA and have been shown to reduce pain and activity limitations in this group of patients [11, 12, 15].

M. van der Leeden • W. Peter
Amsterdam Rehabilitation Research Center I Reade, Amsterdam, The Netherlands

J. Dekker (✉)
Department of Rehabilitation Medicine, VU University Medical Center, PO Box 7057, 1007 MB Amsterdam, The Netherlands

Department of Psychiatry, VU University Medical Center, Amsterdam, The Netherlands
e-mail: j.dekker@vumc.nl

J. Dekker (ed.), *Exercise and Physical Functioning in Osteoarthritis: Medical, Neuromuscular and Behavioral Perspectives*, Springer Briefs in Specialty Topics in Behavioral Medicine, DOI 10.1007/978-1-4614-7215-5_7, © The Author(s) 2014

The focus in muscle strengthening exercises is primarily on two types of muscle function. Muscular *strength* is the maximum amount of force a muscle or muscle group can generate. Muscular *endurance* is the ability of the muscles to sustain muscle action (a repeated action or a single static action). Low repetition, high resistance training enhances *strength* development, whereas high repetition, low-intensity training optimizes muscular *endurance* [16]. Exercises should be performed 2–3 days a week on alternate days, using resistance adequate to induce fatigue [17]. For knee and hip OA patients, muscle strengthening exercises focus mainly on the quadriceps, hamstrings, and glutei muscles.

Strength gains are highly specific to the movement patterns used in training. For maximum benefit, a resistant or weight-bearing training program should include activities quite similar to those experienced as problematic in patient's daily life. For example, *strength* is needed to step on a high surface (e.g., getting into a bus or train), whereas *endurance* of the muscles is needed for walking the stairs several times a day. Thus, depending on the activity limitations experienced in daily life, the content of the muscle strengthening training program should be established.

Aerobic Exercises

Aerobic exercises are aimed at improvement of the aerobic capacity, meaning an improvement of the condition of the heart and lungs needed for an optimal oxygen uptake of the muscles. In addition, improved circulation by aerobic exercises increases nutrition of the muscles and thereby decreases muscle soreness after training [16].

Performance of aerobic exercises is associated with important health benefits for the general population [1]. In OA patients, it has been shown that aerobic exercises, in combination with muscle strengthening exercises, also reduce pain and activity limitations [11, 12]. To improve aerobic capacity, the American College of Sports Medicine (ACSM) guidelines recommend to exercise for 3–5 days a week at 70–85 % of age-predicted maximal heart rate at a duration on 20–30 min [17]. Examples of aerobic exercises are bicycling, aquatic exercises, and walking. These exercises can be performed safely by persons with symptomatic joints [1], without increasing the risk of progression [18]. High impact exercises, such as sports that require jumping (e.g., basketball, volleyball, and dancing) must be performed with more caution since they may exacerbate pain and increase the risks of injuries [19].

Flexibility Exercises

One of the consequences of OA is limited range of joint motion (ROM) caused by joint stiffness and soft-tissue shortening. Limited ROM may lead to limitations in performing daily activities such as walking [20].

Flexibility exercises consist of ROM exercises and active stretching exercises. ROM exercises are exercises in which the joint is taken in its full available range for several times without holding the end position. In stretching exercises, gentle and controlled tension is set on the targeted soft tissues and hold in the maximum possible position [16]. Stretching exercises can be performed both actively (by the patient itself) and passively (by the therapist). The ACSM guidelines recommend to stretch for 10–30 s, 3–4 repetitions for each stretch, with a minimum frequency of 2–3 days a week [17].

The effectiveness of isolated flexibility exercises in knee and hip OA has scarcely been studied. In an RCT, the effect of a manual therapy program on hip function was found to be superior to an exercise therapy program with active and passive stretching in patients with OA of the hip. Manual therapy is particularly aimed at the improvement of elasticity of the joint capsule and the surrounding muscles and includes manipulation and stretching techniques. Patients in the manual therapy group had significantly better outcomes on pain, stiffness, hip function, and ROM, although the exercise therapy group also improved on these outcomes [21].

Thus, flexibility exercises may lead to an increase in joint ROM and, in combination with other exercises, to a reduction of pain and activity limitations in knee and hip OA. However, more research is needed to establish the effect of flexibility exercises in OA patients.

Functional Exercises

Common activities that are limited in patients with hip and knee OA include walking, stair climbing, rising up, and sitting down from a chair or bed and getting in and out of a car. To improve activities in daily living, it is supposed to be important to train the activities itself, besides training of functions related to these activities such as muscle function, aerobic capacity, and flexibility [22]. An adequate performance of activities is not the product of the individual functions but the integration of these functions in a certain activity (http://www.who.int/classifications/icf/en).

The level of difficulty of functional exercises can be increased during the treatment period. For example, if a patient has problems climbing the stairs, the first step in the functional training can be stepping on a small height. In the next steps, the height can be increased as well as the frequency of stepping. In the final step, the activity itself (stair climbing) in the patient's own environment can be practiced. Another example is functional training for a patient experiencing walking problems. First, walking exercises can be performed inside on a flat underground. Subsequently, different undergrounds can be used with increasing difficulty; outdoors, on sand, in a forest, etc. Finally, the walking distance can be extended, eventually leading to a better walking performance in daily life.

In conclusion, functional exercises should be an essential component of exercise therapy in order to reduce patient-specific activity limitations in knee and hip OA. Physical therapists play a crucial role in the assessment of activity limitations and should adjust the exercise program accordingly.

Exercise Delivery and Adherence

Exercises can be performed individually or in a group, with or without supervision of a physical therapist. The effect of group exercises compared with individual exercises has not been studied in OA. Supervised exercises were found to be superior over home exercises in two studies with good methodological quality [23, 24].

As adherence appears to be an important factor in long-term outcome from exercise in knee and hip OA, strategies to improve adherence have been adopted such as long-term monitoring [19]. Long-term effects on pain and activity limitations were found in several RCTs in which additional booster sessions after the period of exercise therapy were given [25]. Similarly, it seems of great importance to encourage patients to start recreational activities or sport after the period of exercise therapy. However, some activities are likely to be harmful in the long term, particularly those that involve high velocity impact (e.g., jumping and running) on an already-injured joint surface; thus these should be discouraged [19]. Bicycling, walking, and aquatic exercise are supposed to be safe for patients with knee and hip OA.

Duration, Frequency, and Intensity of Exercises

Limited evidence is available for the optimal duration, frequency, and intensity of exercises in knee and hip OA. With regard to the number of treatment sessions, the only evidence comprises a comparison in the Cochrane review for knee OA between the effect of treatment programs of less than 12 sessions and more than 12 sessions [11]. This comparison demonstrated a higher effect on activity limitations for the program with more than 12 sessions. Similarly, little is known about the optimal intensity and frequency of exercises in knee and hip OA. Only one study compared the effect of high intensive cycling training with low intensive cycling training on outcome in knee OA patients. No differences between the groups were found in functional ability, pain, gait, and aerobic capacity [26, 27]. Further research concerning the optimal duration, intensity, and frequency of exercises in knee and hip OA is recommended.

In view of the heterogeneity of the group of OA patients, tailoring of exercises to the characteristics of the individual patient seems important. To increase the effect and to guarantee safety, physical therapists should be involved in the development and evaluation of the exercise program, especially in patients with complex health problems (i.e., patients with high pain scores, a high level of activity limitations and/or comorbidities).

Conclusion

Regular exercises in OA comprise exercises aiming at improvement of muscle strength, aerobic capacity, flexibility, and daily weight-bearing activities. These exercises have been found to be effective in reducing pain and activity limitations in knee OA and are most likely to be effective in hip OA. The ACSM guidelines provide preliminary guidance for determining the duration, frequency, and intensity of an exercise program. However, more research is needed concerning the optimal duration, intensity, and frequency of exercises in knee and hip OA. To increase the effect and to guarantee safety, physical therapists should be involved in the development and evaluation of an exercise program, especially in OA patients with complex health problems. Furthermore, it is recommended that a supervised exercise period is followed by booster sessions to preserve the achieved effect. Encouragement to be physically active should be incorporated in these booster sessions.

In addition to regular exercises, it may be necessary to target exercises to specific patient characteristics to increase the effect of the exercise program. Recent research suggests an important role of knee joint stabilization and avoidance of activities in the development of activity limitations (Chaps. 5 and 6). Chapters 8 and 9 describe current evidence for exercise therapy targeting these factors.

References

1. Westby MD, Minor MA (2006) Exercise and physical activity. In: Bartlett SJ, Bingham CO, Maricic MJ, Daly Iversen M, Ruffing V (eds) Clinical care in the rheumatic diseases, 3rd edn. Atlanta, Association of Rheumatology Health Professionals, pp 211–220
2. American College of Rheumatology Subcommittee on Osteoarthritis Guidelines (2000) Recommendations for the medical management of osteoarthritis of the hip and knee: 2000 update. Arthritis Rheum 43(9):1905–1915
3. Jordan KM, Arden NK, Doherty M, Bannwarth B, Bijlsma JW, Dieppe P et al (2003) EULAR Recommendations 2003: an evidence based approach to the management of knee osteoarthritis: report of a Task Force of the Standing Committee for International Clinical Studies Including Therapeutic Trials (ESCISIT). Ann Rheum Dis 62(12):1145–1155
4. Conaghan PG, Dickson J, Grant RL (2008) Care and management of osteoarthritis in adults: summary of NICE guidance. BMJ 336(7642):502–503
5. Zhang W, Doherty M, Arden N, Bannwarth B, Bijlsma J, Gunther KP et al (2005) EULAR evidence based recommendations for the management of hip osteoarthritis: report of a task force of the EULAR Standing Committee for International Clinical Studies Including Therapeutics (ESCISIT). Ann Rheum Dis 64(5):669–681
6. Zhang W, Moskowitz RW, Nuki G, Abramson S, Altman RD, Arden N et al (2008) OARSI recommendations for the management of hip and knee osteoarthritis, part II: OARSI evidence-based, expert consensus guidelines. Osteoarthritis Cartilage 16(2):137–162
7. Zhang W, Moskowitz RW, Nuki G, Abramson S, Altman RD, Arden N et al (2007) OARSI recommendations for the management of hip and knee osteoarthritis, part I: critical appraisal of existing treatment guidelines and systematic review of current research evidence. Osteoarthritis Cartilage 15(9):981–1000

8. Roddy E, Zhang W, Doherty M, Arden NK, Barlow J, Birrell F et al (2005) Evidence-based recommendations for the role of exercise in the management of osteoarthritis of the hip or knee–the MOVE consensus. Rheumatology (Oxford) 44(1):67–73

9. Smidt N, de Vet HC, Bouter LM, Dekker J, Arendzen JH, de Bie RA et al (2005) Effectiveness of exercise therapy: a best-evidence summary of systematic reviews. Aust J Physiother 51(2):71–85

10. van Baar ME, Assendelft WJ, Dekker J, Oostendorp RA, Bijlsma JW (1999) Effectiveness of exercise therapy in patients with osteoarthritis of the hip or knee: a systematic review of randomized clinical trials. Arthritis Rheum 42(7):1361–1369

11. Fransen M, McConnell S (2008) Exercise for osteoarthritis of the knee. Cochrane Database Syst Rev 4:CD004376

12. Fransen M, McConnell S, Bell M (2003) Exercise for osteoarthritis of the hip or knee. Cochrane Database Syst Rev 3:CD004286

13. Dekker J, van Dijk GM, Veenhof C (2009) Risk factors for functional decline in osteoarthritis of the hip or knee. Curr Opin Rheumatol 21(5):520–524

14. van Dijk GM, Dekker J, Veenhof C, van den Ende CH (2006) Course of functional status and pain in osteoarthritis of the hip or knee: a systematic review of the literature. Arthritis Rheum 55(5):779–785

15. van Baar ME, Dekker J, Oostendorp RA, Bijl D, Voorn TB, Bijlsma JW (2001) Effectiveness of exercise in patients with osteoarthritis of hip or knee: nine months' follow up. Ann Rheum Dis 60(12):1123–1130

16. Willmore JH, Costill DL (1994) Physiology of sport and exercise. Human Kinetics, Champaign, IL

17. American College of Sports Medicine (2000) ACSM's guidelines for exercise testing and prescription, 6th edn. Lippincott Williams & Wilkins, Philadelphia, PA

18. Chapple CM, Nicholson H, Baxter GD, Abbott JH (2011) Patient characteristics that predict progression of knee osteoarthritis: a systematic review of prognostic studies. Arthritis Care Res (Hoboken) 63(8):1115–1125

19. Hunter DJ, Eckstein F (2009) Exercise and osteoarthritis. J Anat 214(2):197–207

20. Steultjens MP, Dekker J, van Baar ME, Oostendorp RA, Bijlsma JW (2000) Range of joint motion and disability in patients with osteoarthritis of the knee or hip. Rheumatology (Oxford) 39(9):955–961

21. Hoeksma HL, Dekker J, Ronday HK, Heering A, van der Lubbe N, Vel C et al (2004) Comparison of manual therapy and exercise therapy in osteoarthritis of the hip: a randomized clinical trial. Arthritis Rheum 51(5):722–729

22. Peter WF, Jansen MJ, Hurkmans EJ, Bloo H, Dekker J, Dilling RG et al (2011) Physiotherapy in hip and knee osteoarthritis: development of a practice guideline concerning initial assessment, treatment and evaluation. Acta Reumatol Port 36(3):268–281

23. Deyle GD, Allison SC, Matekel RL, Ryder MG, Stang JM, Gohdes DD et al (2005) Physical therapy treatment effectiveness for osteoarthritis of the knee: a randomized comparison of supervised clinical exercise and manual therapy procedures versus a home exercise program. Phys Ther 85(12):1301–1317

24. McCarthy CJ, Mills PM, Pullen R, Roberts C, Silman A, Oldham JA (2004) Supplementing a home exercise programme with a class-based exercise programme is more effective than home exercise alone in the treatment of knee osteoarthritis. Rheumatology (Oxford) 43(7):880–886

25. Pisters MF, Veenhof C, Schellevis FG, Twisk JW, Dekker J, de Bakker DH (2010) Exercise adherence improving long-term patient outcome in patients with osteoarthritis of the hip and/or knee. Arthritis Care Res (Hoboken) 62(8):1087–1094

26. Mangione KK, McCully K, Gloviak A, Lefebvre I, Hofmann M, Craik R (1999) The effects of high-intensity and low-intensity cycle ergometry in older adults with knee osteoarthritis. J Gerontol A Biol Sci Med Sci 54(4):M184–M190

27. Brosseau L, MacLeay L, Robinson V, Wells G, Tugwell P (2003) Intensity of exercise for the treatment of osteoarthritis. Cochrane Database Syst Rev 2:CD004259

Chapter 8
Exercise Therapy Targeting Neuromuscular Mechanisms

Jesper Knoop, Martijn P.M. Steultjens, and Joost Dekker

Exercise therapy is effective in patients with knee OA. In national [1] and international guidelines for the treatment of knee OA [2–4], exercise therapy is recommended. Exercise therapy predominantly aims to improve lower extremity muscle strength. However, as mentioned in Chap. 7, only moderate effects of exercise therapy in reducing pain and activity limitations have been demonstrated at best [5]. Some persons do not seem to benefit from exercising. This suggests that innovative exercise modalities need to be developed, not only targeting muscle weakness, but also other, more specific mechanisms of activity limitations, for instance neuromuscular mechanisms.

In this chapter, we first discuss the rationale of such innovative exercise modalities that target neuromuscular mechanisms for patients with OA. Second, an overview of different modalities of exercise therapy targeting neuromuscular mechanisms and three examples of specific programs will be provided. Finally, we summarize available evidence for the effectiveness of exercise therapy targeting neuromuscular mechanisms in patients with OA and provide suggestions for future work.

J. Knoop
Amsterdam Rehabilitation Research Center | Reade, Amsterdam, The Netherlands

M.P.M. Steultjens
School of Health and Life Sciences, Institute for Applied Health Research
Glasgow Caledonian University, Glasgow, Lanarkshire, UK

J. Dekker (✉)
Department of Rehabilitation Medicine, VU University Medical Center, PO Box 7057,
1007 MB Amsterdam, The Netherlands

Department of Psychiatry, VU University Medical Center, Amsterdam, The Netherlands
e-mail: j.dekker@vumc.nl

J. Dekker (ed.), *Exercise and Physical Functioning in Osteoarthritis: Medical,*
Neuromuscular and Behavioral Perspectives, Springer Briefs in Specialty Topics in
Behavioral Medicine, DOI 10.1007/978-1-4614-7215-5_8, © The Author(s) 2014

Rationale

Lower limb muscle strength, proprioceptive acuity, and the passive restraint system (i.e., ligaments and capsule of joint) of the knee joint are considered to be essential for neuromuscular control of the knee [6–8]. Unfortunately, these factors can be impaired in OA. A lack of neuromuscular control may cause instability of the joint, which is experienced as a feeling of buckling, shifting, or giving way. Recurrent episodes of instability may result in activity limitations [7–9]. To counteract instability, it is crucial that therapy focuses on factors involved in neuromuscular control.

In Chap. 5, it has been discussed that muscle strength alone, although a crucial factor for joint stabilization, may not always be sufficient to maintain stability of the joint. Poor proprioception, varus–valgus laxity (due to impaired passive restraint system) and high varus–valgus motion of the knee joint during walking were found to aggravate the impact of lower limb muscle weakness on activity limitations [10–12]. This could imply that in the presence of poor proprioception, laxity, or high knee motion during walking, muscle strengthening exercises may not be sufficient to improve the performance of activities. Muscle strengthening of the lower extremity may not result in improvements in performance of daily activities, if neuromuscular control remains inadequate. Exercise therapy may therefore need to target other factors involved in neuromuscular control, in addition to muscle weakness. Furthermore, in order to perform high-intensity strengthening exercises effectively and safely without risking knee injuries, adequate neuromuscular control might be essential. This implies that neuromuscular exercises need to precede strengthening exercises. To conclude, exercise may need to target poor proprioception, laxity, and varus–valgus knee motion in the first phase of treatment in order to optimize neuromuscular control of the knee. When this has been achieved, traditional muscle strengthening exercises can be added in the second phase. We discuss this rationale in more detail below.

First Phase: Neuromuscular Training

In the first phase of the exercise program, neuromuscular training is provided. Exercises aim at improving proprioceptive acuity, limiting the consequences of impaired passive restraint system (laxity), and minimizing varus–valgus movements of the joint. Quality of exercise performance is critical during neuromuscular training. Exercise intensity and difficulty can only be increased, when quality of exercise performance can be sustained.

Two components of proprioception can be distinguished (1) the sensation or awareness of joint motion or position in space and (2) the ability to actively control joint motion or position. Both components of proprioceptive acuity can be trained, in which the first might be required to improve the second. First, a patient needs to become aware of the position and movements of the knee during exercising as well as during performance of daily activities. If awareness is improved, exercises can also target the ability to actively control movements of the joint.

Enhanced proprioception, i.e., awareness and adequate control of knee position, is also presumed to reduce the consequences of impaired passive restraint system, i.e., laxity. In lax joints, sudden unintended movements of the joint may occur. Since the structures involved in the passive restraint system (i.e., ligament and capsule) are not presumed to be modifiable, compensating strategies are required such as optimal awareness of movements of the joint and actively controlling joint position by adequate muscle use.

Finally, the amount of varus–valgus (sideways) motion of the knee during walking might be minimized by instructing the patient to focus on maintaining neutral alignment of the knee joint, i.e., keeping the hip–knee–ankle joints in a straight line, which corresponds to a neutral loading pattern of the knee joint. This means that patients need to prevent varus and valgus malalignment during exercising and in daily life. For this purpose, adequate proprioception and active muscle control are necessary.

Second Phase: Muscle Strengthening Training

Muscle strengthening may only result in improvements in performance of daily activities when neuromuscular control has been enhanced sufficiently. Furthermore, neuromuscular control is presumed to be essential for adequate and safe performance of higher-intensity strengthening exercises. Therefore, neuromuscular training is provided in the first phase, while muscle strengthening exercises are given in the second phase. Muscle strengthening exercises can be gradually increased in intensity. It is important to maintain neuromuscular control during the program. This implies that in the second phase, exercises not only aim at muscle strengthening but also focuses on neuromuscular mechanisms.

Modalities

Several programs for neuromuscular training have been developed. The basic principle of neuromuscular training is that repetitively challenging an individual's ability to maintain static or dynamic control of knee joint results in enhanced neuromuscular control and subsequently in improved knee stability [13].

Neuromuscular training can be subdivided into four different modalities.

(a) General proprioceptive exercises
(b) Balance and perturbation exercises
(c) Agility exercises
(d) Functional neuromuscular training

We discuss each of these four modalities briefly. Additionally, we provide three examples of exercise programs that are specifically developed to improve neuromuscular control. In each of these programs, all four modalities are incorporated.

General Proprioceptive Exercises

Proprioceptive exercises are coordinative exercises that specifically focus on a patient's ability to control and position the knee accurately. For this purpose, instructions from the therapist and feedback by a mirror on knee position can be provided. An example of a proprioceptive exercise is a "lunge" (forward) step, in which a patient is instructed to stand in this position for a few seconds, while maintaining knee position in line with ankle and hip (i.e., neutral alignment), avoiding knee-over-toe position; the patient is instructed to prevent the knee from buckling, giving way or shifting (see Fig. 8.1). Proprioceptive exercises can be first provided under nonweight-bearing circumstances (hydrotherapy or exercises in sitting position), while dynamic weight-bearing exercises are given at a later stage.

Recently, a computer program for proprioceptive exercises has been developed [14]. With this computer program, a patient is instructed to move a cursor on the computer screen by moving his feet or leg in that direction, while not looking directly at his legs. The patient receives feedback during this exercise from the computer screen.

Balance and Perturbation Training

Balance training focuses on postural control during standing. Examples of balance exercises are standing on one leg, standing with eyes closed, walking over a line, or walking on a soft unstable surface. Perturbation training is balance training incorporating the use of roller boards or wobble boards. This training modality is frequently used in patients with knee injuries, for instance anterior cruciate ligament rupture [15]. Complexity of the exercise can be increased by providing double tasks like counting or starting a conversation during the exercise. Three examples of balance and perturbation training are provided in Fig. 8.2.

Agility Training

Agility training involves quick stops and starts, cutting and turning, and changes in direction to expose patients to activities that challenge the knee to potentially

0

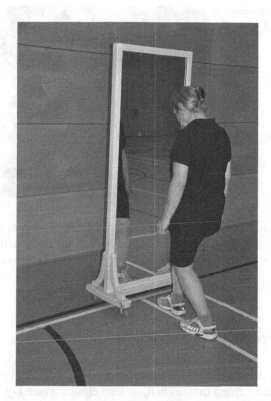

Fig. 8.1 Lunge (forward step) in front of a mirror, focusing on neutral alignment of hip–knee–ankle

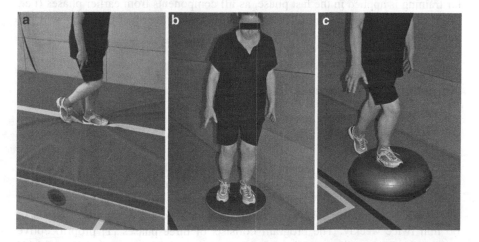

Fig. 8.2 Three examples of balance and perturbation training (**a**) walking on soft unstable surface, (**b**) standing balance on wobble board, and (**c**) "lunge" step on soft unstable surface

Fig. 8.3 Functional training of stair climbing and descending

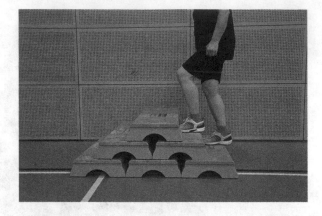

destabilizing loads. These exercises may help patients to learn to deal with potentially destabilizing loads when encountered in regular daily activities [15]. For more challenging agility training, similar exercises can be provided on unstable surfaces.

Functional Neuromuscular Training

In this modality, daily activities are trained that are relevant and problematic for a patient, like walking, rising from a chair, or stair climbing (see Fig. 8.3). Functional neuromuscular training aims at maintaining knee stability during these activities. Episodes of knee instability mostly occur during walking [7], therefore gait training is the main component of this modality. In most programs, functional neuromuscular training is applied in the last phase, as all components from earlier phases (i.e., proprioceptive training, muscle strengthening, and aerobic training) will be integrated in this modality.

Neuromuscular Exercise Programs

STABILITY-Program

The STABILITY-program is an exercise program that specifically focuses on neuromuscular mechanisms. The program has recently been developed in the Netherlands for knee OA patients with instability of the knee joint. The STABILTY-program is a 12-week program with supervised training sessions of 60 min twice weekly. The program consists of three phases [1] proprioceptive training in the first phase [2], muscle strengthening in the second phase, and [3] training of daily activities in the third phase (see Fig. 8.4). Each of these phases will be described below.

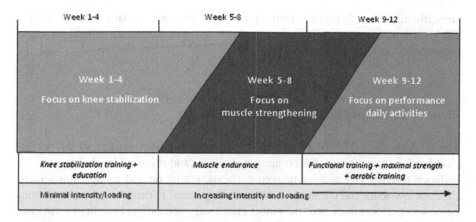

Fig. 8.4 Overview of STABILITY-program

Phase 1: Proprioceptive Training (Weeks 1–4)

In the first phase, exercises aim at improving the patient's awareness of and control over lower extremity movements, in particular movements of the knee. The physical therapist specifically focuses on neuromuscular control during exercises, by:

(a) Instructing the patient to look at his knees by promoting use of visual feedback (by using a mirror)
(b) Instructing the patient to focus on knee position by promoting use of proprioceptive stimuli
(c) Providing tactile feedback on knee position by manually moving a patient's knee in a neutrally aligned position
(d) Providing verbal feedback to the patient on knee position
(e) Continuously reminding the patient of the importance of focusing on controlled performance of movements and neutral alignment
(f) Encouraging patients to perform exercises in a controlled fashion

In this first phase, only low-intensity exercises are provided. In the first week, sessions are performed in a swimming pool, to minimize knee loading during exercising. General education on osteoarthritis, information on the management of the condition, and the rationale for the STABILITY-approach are provided in the first phase as well.

Phase 2: Muscle Strengthening (Weeks 5–8)

In the second phase of the STABILITY-program, the focus shifts from neuromuscular training to muscle strengthening. The intensity of exercises and joint loading is gradually increased each week but remains submaximal, with fatigue as primary indicator of adequate intensity level. Although the focus has shifted to muscle strengthening, the therapist's instructions and feedback remain focused on the controlled performance of knee movements and on patient awareness of these movements during the exercises.

Phase 3: Functional Training (Weeks 9–12)

The final phase of STABILITY-program mainly comprises training of the performance of daily activities, which are problematic and relevant for the patient, for instance walking (on even or uneven surface), sitting on and rising from a chair (high or low seat), and climbing and descending stairs. Patients receive instructions on how to perform these activities most effectively and safely. Stability of the knee has to be maintained during these activities. Muscle strengthening and aerobic exercises are provided in addition to this functional training. Intensity of exercises is gradually increased to the highest possible level; the (in)ability to perform an exercise due to insufficient strength is the primary indicator for adequate intensity level. However, therapist instructions and feedback remain focused on the quality of exercise performance. Patients are encouraged to remain physically active in daily life after completing the exercise program.

NEMEX Training Program

Another example of an exercise program targeting neuromuscular mechanisms is the NEuroMuscular Exercise training program (NEMEX) [16]. This program has been developed in Sweden for patients with severe knee or hip OA waiting for total knee arthroplasty. The NEMEX-program is a supervised exercise program with sessions of 60 min twice weekly. The number of weeks of training is approximately 12 weeks, depending on the length of the waiting list for surgery. Each training session consists of three parts: a 10-min warming-up (ergometer cycle), a 40-min circuit program, consisting of training of core stability/postural function, postural orientation, lower extremity muscle strength and functional exercises, and a 10-min cooling down (walking/stretching). Physical therapists supervising the sessions emphasize the quality of the performance, by instructing the patient to achieve neutral alignment of the lower limb, i.e., with the hip, knee, and foot well aligned. When an exercise is adequately performed in a controlled manner and with minimal exertion, progression in exercise intensity and difficulty can be achieved by increasing the number of repetitions, varying the direction and velocity of the movements, increasing the load, and/or changing the support surface. See Ageberg et al. [16] for more detailed information.

Neuromuscular Program for Early OA

A third example is a neuromuscular exercise program, which has been developed in Sweden for patients with early signs of knee OA [17]. This exercise program consists of two supervised sessions a week for 8 weeks, aiming at improving lower extremity strength and neuromuscular control. Primary aim of the program is to minimize knee joint loading. Each training session consists of a 10-min warming-up (ergometer cycle or treadmill), four stations of neuromuscular and hip/knee strengthening exercises, and stretching exercises for lower extremity muscles. Exercises are performed with sustained neuromuscular control, i.e., without sudden changes in speed or direction. Furthermore, patients are instructed to maintain neutral knee alignment throughout all exercises. Exercise intensity is increased when exercises can be easily performed, i.e., without losing quality of performance. Only if pain exceeds the level which the patient judges as acceptable or if increased pain symptoms persist after 24 h, intensity will be lowered. Patients are encouraged to maintain neutral knee alignment during physical activities in daily life and to perform weight bearing, submaximal activities, such as walking, or aerobics, for at least 30 min every day. See Thorstensson et al. [17] for more detailed information.

Evidence for Effectiveness of Neuromuscular Exercise Therapy

Exercise programs targeting neuromuscular mechanisms for knee OA patients have been developed only recently. Therefore, limited evidence on the effectiveness of these programs is available. Below, we summarize the existing evidence.

It is well known that exercise therapy has a beneficial effect on muscle strength. Also proprioception can be improved by exercise therapy [18]. Several explanations for the effects of exercising on proprioceptive acuity can be offered. First, it is hypothesized that exercise increases mechanoreceptor sensitivity (muscle spindle sensitivity in particular) [18]. Second, by increasing muscle mass, exercise therapy might be able to increase the number of muscle spindle units [19]. Finally, exercise therapy may reduce muscle fatigue and muscle contraction [19], which has a positive effect on proprioceptive acuity [20, 21]. It is unknown which type of exercises is most effective in improving proprioceptive acuity [22, 23], except for a superiority of weight-bearing over nonweight-bearing exercises [24]. This superiority might be explained by the increase in intra-articular pressure, which plays a role in the sensitivity of Ruffini nerve endings [24].

The effect of exercise on neuromuscular factors, other than muscle strength and proprioception, has not been evaluated. The passive restraint system, i.e., ligaments and capsule, is not presumed to be modifiable by exercising, while the effect on varus–valgus knee motion during activities is unknown.

Ageberg et al. [16] determined the feasibility of their neuromuscular exercise program (NEMEX) in an uncontrolled pilot study. A total of 66 patients, scheduled for total hip or knee replacement, participated in the study. The authors of this study concluded that the NEMEX program was feasible in patients with severe knee OA. Thorstensson et al. [17] investigated the effect of a 8-week exercise program of neuromuscular and strengthening exercises on peak knee loading, in a uncontrolled pilot study in 13 patients with early signs of knee OA. The program was found be effective in reducing knee loading, but only during one-leg rising and not during gait. Both studies pointed out that neuromuscular exercise programs can have positive results. However, because no comparison was made with traditional exercise therapy, conclusions on superiority of neuromuscular exercises over traditional exercises cannot be drawn. In contrast to these two studies, a research group from Taiwan compared computerized proprioceptive exercises with strengthening exercises, demonstrating similar effects of both programs [23]. Superiority of proprioceptive training could not be demonstrated.

Three recent studies evaluated the combination of neuromuscular and muscle strengthening exercises, in comparison to muscle strengthening exercises only [25, 26]. Firstly, Diracoglu et al. [25, 27] compared an experimental program consisting of kinesthesia (proprioceptive), balance, and strengthening exercises with a control program consisting of muscle strengthening exercises only. Both programs consisted of 24 supervised sessions in an 8-week period. Sixty female participants were alternately allocated to either the experimental or the control group in order of admission to the clinic (i.e., not at random). Both exercise programs were found to be effective, with significantly better effects in the experimental group on self-reported activity limitations but not on self-reported pain. Group differences on activity limitations were only small and presumably not clinically meaningful. Remarkably, proprioceptive improvements were found to be similar in the groups. Training intensity was higher in the experimental intervention, which possibly explains the group differences [27]. Because of the study limitations, the study does not allow distinct conclusions. Secondly, in a larger randomized controlled trial by Fitzgerald et al. [26], 183 knee OA patients were treated with an experimental treatment of agility, perturbation, and muscle strengthening exercises or with a control treatment of muscle strengthening exercises only. Both exercise programs consisted of 12 supervised sessions in a 6–8-week period. Although both groups exhibited improvements in self-reported activity limitations as well as in other outcomes, there were no differences between groups. A limitation of this study is that only one-third of the participants reported instability of the knee at inclusion, while two-thirds did not. This may have limited the power of the study to demonstrate superior effectiveness of the combination of neuromuscular and traditional exercise therapy. Thirdly, the effectiveness of a neuromuscular exercise program, specifically targeting knee stabilization, in combination with muscle strengthening and functional exercises (i.e., STABILITY-program, described in previous section) has been evaluated by our study group [28]. In this randomized controlled trial, we specifically selected knee OA patients with instability of the knee joint ($n = 159$) who were randomized over two groups:

the experimental group ($n = 80$) receiving the STABILITY-program and the control group ($n = 79$) receiving muscle strengthening and functional exercises only, for 12 weeks with two sessions a week. Although the STABILITY-program was found to be highly effective in reducing activity limitations (30 % improvement), pain (40 % improvement), and self-reported knee stability (30 % improvement), no additional effect could be demonstrated compared to the control program. These findings, together with the studies by Diracoglu et al. and Fitzgerald et al., are indicative for a dominant role of muscle function in knee stabilization and highlight the importance of exercises targeting muscle strength in patients with knee OA, also in those with instability of the knee joint.

Studies on the effectiveness of neuromuscular exercises have only been performed in patients with knee OA, while not in hip OA. Although it can be presumed that neuromuscular mechanisms in knee OA patients also apply to hip OA, specific programs have not been developed for this group of patients so far.

In conclusion, a limited number of studies evaluated the effectiveness of exercise therapy aiming at neuromuscular mechanisms in knee OA, while none of them in hip OA. Neuromuscular exercise seems to be effective in reducing pain and activity limitations. The additional effect of exercises targeting neuromuscular mechanisms over traditional muscle strengthening programs has not been demonstrated yet.

References

1. Peter WF, Jansen MJ, Hurkmans EJ, Bloo H, Dekker J, Dilling RG et al (2011) Physiotherapy in hip and knee osteoarthritis: development of a practice guideline concerning initial assessment, treatment and evaluation. Acta Reumatol Port 36(3):268–281
2. Zhang W, Nuki G, Moskowitz RW, Abramson S, Altman RD, Arden NK et al (2010) OARSI recommendations for the management of hip and knee osteoarthritis: part III: changes in evidence following systematic cumulative update of research published through January 2009. Osteoarthritis Cartilage 18(4):476–499
3. Hochberg MC, Altman RD, April KT, Benkhalti M, Guyatt G, McGowan J et al (2012) American College of Rheumatology 2012 recommendations for the use of nonpharmacologic and pharmacologic therapies in osteoarthritis of the hand, hip, and knee. Arthritis Care Res (Hoboken) 64(4):455–474
4. Jordan KM, Arden NK, Doherty M, Bannwarth B, Bijlsma JW, Dieppe P et al (2003) EULAR recommendations 2003: an evidence based approach to the management of knee osteoarthritis: report of a Task Force of the Standing Committee for International Clinical Studies Including Therapeutic Trials (ESCISIT). Ann Rheum Dis 62(12):1145–1155
5. Fransen M, McConnell S (2008) Exercise for osteoarthritis of the knee. Cochrane Database Syst Rev 4:CD004376
6. Fitzgerald GK, Piva SR, Irrgang JJ (2004) Reports of joint instability in knee osteoarthritis: its prevalence and relationship to physical function. Arthritis Rheum 51(6):941–946
7. Knoop J, van der Leeden M, van der Esch M, Thorstensson CA, Gerritsen M, Voorneman RE et al (2012) Association of lower muscle strength with self-reported knee instability in osteoarthritis of the knee: results from the Amsterdam Osteoarthritis Cohort. Arthritis Care Res (Hoboken) 64(1):38–45

8. Schmitt LC, Fitzgerald GK, Reisman AS, Rudolph KS (2008) Instability, laxity, and physical function in patients with medial knee osteoarthritis. Phys Ther 88(12):1506–1516

9. Felson DT, Niu J, McClennan C, Sack B, Aliabadi P, Hunter DJ et al (2007) Knee buckling: prevalence, risk factors, and associated limitations in function. Ann Intern Med 147 (8):534–540

10. van der Esch M, Steultjens M, Harlaar J, Knol D, Lems W, Dekker J (2007) Joint proprioception, muscle strength, and functional ability in patients with osteoarthritis of the knee. Arthritis Rheum 57(5):787–793

11. van der Esch M, Steultjens M, Knol DL, Dinant H, Dekker J (2006) Joint laxity and the relationship between muscle strength and functional ability in patients with osteoarthritis of the knee. Arthritis Rheum 55(6):953–959

12. van der Esch M, Steultjens M, Harlaar J, Wolterbeek N, Knol D, Dekker J (2008) Varus-valgus motion and functional ability in patients with knee osteoarthritis. Ann Rheum Dis 67 (4):471–477

13. Williams GN, Chmielewski T, Rudolph K, Buchanan TS, Snyder-Mackler L (2001) Dynamic knee stability: current theory and implications for clinicians and scientists. J Orthop Sports Phys Ther 31(10):546–566

14. Jan MH, Tang PF, Lin JJ, Tseng SC, Lin YF, Lin DH (2008) Efficacy of a target-matching foot-stepping exercise on proprioception and function in patients with knee osteoarthritis. J Orthop Sports Phys Ther 38(1):19–25

15. Fitzgerald GK, Childs JD, Ridge TM, Irrgang JJ (2002) Agility and perturbation training for a physically active individual with knee osteoarthritis. Phys Ther 82(4):372–382

16. Ageberg E, Link A, Roos EM (2010) Feasibility of neuromuscular training in patients with severe hip or knee OA: the individualized goal-based NEMEX-TJR training program. BMC Musculoskelet Disord 11:126

17. Thorstensson CA, Henriksson M, von Porat A, Sjodahl C, Roos EM (2007) The effect of eight weeks of exercise on knee adduction moment in early knee osteoarthritis–a pilot study. Osteoarthritis Cartilage 15(10):1163–1170

18. Knoop J, Steultjens MP, van der Leeden M, van der Esch M, Thorstensson CA, Roorda LD et al (2011) Proprioception in knee osteoarthritis: a narrative review. Osteoarthritis Cartilage 19(4):381–388

19. Butler AA, Lord SR, Rogers MW, Fitzpatrick RC (2008) Muscle weakness impairs the proprioceptive control of human standing. Brain Res 1242:244–251

20. Wise AK, Gregory JE, Proske U (1998) Detection of movements of the human forearm during and after co-contractions of muscles acting at the elbow joint. J Physiol 508(Pt 1):325–330

21. Givoni NJ, Pham T, Allen TJ, Proske U (2007) The effect of quadriceps muscle fatigue on position matching at the knee. J Physiol 584(Pt 1):111–119

22. Lin DH, Lin YF, Chai HM, Han YC, Jan MH (2007) Comparison of proprioceptive functions between computerized proprioception facilitation exercise and closed kinetic chain exercise in patients with knee osteoarthritis. Clin Rheumatol 26(4):520–528

23. Lin DH, Lin CH, Lin YF, Jan MH (2009) Efficacy of 2 non-weight-bearing interventions, proprioception training versus strength training, for patients with knee osteoarthritis: a randomized clinical trial. J Orthop Sports Phys Ther 39(6):450–457

24. Jan MH, Lin CH, Lin YF, Lin JJ, Lin DH (2009) Effects of weight-bearing versus nonweight-bearing exercise on function, walking speed, and position sense in participants with knee osteoarthritis: a randomized controlled trial. Arch Phys Med Rehabil 90(6):897–904

25. Diracoglu D, Aydin R, Baskent A, Celik A (2005) Effects of kinesthesia and balance exercises in knee osteoarthritis. J Clin Rheumatol 11(6):303–310

26. Fitzgerald GK, Piva SR, Gil AB, Wisniewski SR, Oddis CV, Irrgang JJ (2011) Agility and perturbation training techniques in exercise therapy for reducing pain and improving function in people with knee osteoarthritis: a randomized clinical trial. Phys Ther 91(4):452–469

27. Diracoglu D, Baskent A, Celik A, Issever H, Aydin R (2008) Long-term effects of kinesthesia/
    balance and strengthening exercises on patients with knee osteoarthritis: a one-year follow-up
    study. J Back Musculoskelet Rehabil 21(4):253–262
28. Knoop J, Dekker J, Leeden vd M, Esch vd M, Thorstensson CA, Gerritsen M et al (2013) Knee
    joint stabilization therapy in patients with osteoarthritis of the knee: a randomized, controlled
    trial. Osteoarthritis Cartilage (accepted for publication)

Chapter 9
Exercise Aiming at Behavioral Mechanisms

Cindy Veenhof, Martijn Pisters, and Joost Dekker

Exercise therapy in osteoarthritis (OA) of the knee and hip has beneficial effects in the short term. However, the effects seem to decline over time after discharge and finally disappear in the long term [1]. Low exercise adherence rate is seen as one of the main reasons for poor long-term effectiveness of exercise therapy. Furthermore, stimulation of a physical active lifestyle seems important, since a lack of regular physical activity is an important risk factor for functional decline in patients with OA [2] (as described in Chap. 4). A lack of physical activity is partly caused by the avoidance behavior of patients with OA who experience pain during activities. Avoidance behavior is strengthened by negative affect (e.g., anxiety and depression) (see Chap. 6).

Taking this in consideration, it is seems not sufficient to target exercise therapy solely at improvement of impairments (e.g., muscle strength or range of joint motion). Psychological or behavioral oriented interventions such as strategies to improve pain coping and cognitive behavioral therapy can influence psychological distress, pain, and activity limitations [3, 4]. Also, access to information, education, and self-management approaches are included as core elements in the current guidelines [5, 6]. Such approaches are known to improve self-efficacy, anxiety, and depression [7].

Therefore, to enhance long-term effectiveness of exercise therapy, integration of behavioral and/or self-management strategies into exercise therapy treatments seems

C. Veenhof
Netherlands Institute for Health Services Research (NIVEL), Utrecht, The Netherlands

M. Pisters
Clinical Health Sciences, University Medical Center Utrecht, Utrecht, The Netherlands

J. Dekker (✉)
Department of Rehabilitation Medicine, VU University Medical Center, PO Box 7057, 1007 MB Amsterdam, The Netherlands

Department of Psychiatry, VU University Medical Center, Amsterdam, The Netherlands
e-mail: j.dekker@vumc.nl

J. Dekker (ed.), *Exercise and Physical Functioning in Osteoarthritis: Medical, Neuromuscular and Behavioral Perspectives*, Springer Briefs in Specialty Topics in Behavioral Medicine, DOI 10.1007/978-1-4614-7215-5_9, © The Author(s) 2014

a promising approach. In the last years, several of these integrated interventions have been developed and studied in patients with OA of hip and/or knee. Three programs are presented in this chapter to illustrate interventions, which integrate exercise therapy with behavioral or self-management mechanisms.

Exercise Integrated with Behavioral or Self-Management Mechanisms

There are several ways to integrate behavioral or self-management mechanisms in exercise therapy treatment. The following three programs will be described: (1) Behavioral Graded Activity (BGA), an intervention based on the concepts of operant conditioning; (2) Enabling Self-management and Coping with Arthritic knee Pain through Exercise (ESCAPE-knee pain), a cognitive behavioral therapy intervention; and (3) The modified Arthritis Self-Management Program (ASMP), a combination of a self-management program and exercise therapy.

Behavioral Graded Activity

Overview

BGA has been developed by Veenhof et al. [8] and is an individually tailored exercise program for patients with OA. The intervention is directed at increasing the level of activities in a time-contingent way, with the goal to integrate these activities in the daily living of patients. Time-contingency management means that the amount of activities/exercises is based on preset quotas and is not based on pain or other tolerance factors. BGA is based on the concepts of operant conditioning (9, 10). Essential features of the operant conditioning approach are positive reinforcement of healthy behavior, and withdrawal of attention toward pain behavior. The BGA treatment consists of three phases, namely the starting phase (weeks 1–4), treatment phase (weeks 5–12), and integration phase (weeks 13–55). Patients are treated intensively in the first 12 weeks (1 or 2 sessions per week), followed by booster sessions in week 13–55. The duration of each treatment session is approximately 20–30 min.

Content of Intervention

Starting Phase. The starting phase consists of the usual physiotherapy diagnosis, education, selection of activities and exercises, definition of treatment goals, and determination of baseline values. The main educational message in the first weeks of treatment is that physical activity is beneficial (and not harmful) for patients with OA and that avoidance of activities leads to activity limitations. In the starting phase, the patient selects up to three activities, which are most problematic for him or her (e.g., walking, climbing stairs, and gardening). On basis of the patient's impairments and choice of activities, the physiotherapist selects individually tailored exercises to improve impairments (e.g., range of motion and muscle strength). Initial baseline measurements are carried out in which the patient performs and registers the activities. The patient exercises daily at home, to the limit of tolerance (pain contingent), during a week. Next, the patient sets his/her treatment goals for the selected activities. The physiotherapist acts as coach in the goal setting, since it is important that the patient is intrinsically motivated to reach the treatment goal.

Treatment Phase. After the baseline measurements and the goal setting, an individually based scheme is made. In this scheme, the activities (and supporting exercises) will be gradually increased, on a time-contingent basis, to reach the preset goals during the treatment period. Quotas (for endurance time or repetitions) are systematically increased to enable the patient to reach his/her preset goals. To facilitate success experiences at the start of treatment, the quotas start slightly under the mean baseline value. The patient is instructed to perform activities according to the quotas, and not to overperform or underperform the activities. In this way, there is a shift from pain-contingency management during the baseline measurements in the starting phase toward time-contingency management in the treatment phase.

To enhance the patient's motivation, the physiotherapist gives positive reinforcement of physically active behavior and successful completion of the quotas. The patient is advised to continue with his/her activities after the treatment phase. It depends on the goals and the limitations in activities of the individual patient whether the patient is advised to stabilize or to further increase his/her level of activities to a new preset goal.

The gradual increase of activities is only interrupted if an active inflammatory process is suspected or diagnosed (e.g., redness of knee, increase in knee effusion, or comparable symptoms). When the symptoms of an inflammatory process have disappeared, the patient will start again at a lower level of activities. In case of recurrent inflammatory processes, the treatment goals need to be changed as well as the individually based scheme.

Integration Phase. The ultimate goal of BGA is to integrate activities into patients' daily living and, thereby, to increase long-term effectiveness of exercise therapy. However, this behavioral change cannot be performed in a short period of 12 weeks. Therefore, up to seven additional booster sessions are given in the integration phase, respectively in week 18, 25, 34, 42, and 55. During these booster sessions, the patient's activity limitations and adherence to the activities are evaluated. Furthermore, the physiotherapist supports and stimulates the patient to continue with performing the activities and advises him/her how to integrate these in daily living. In case the patient wants to deal with a new problematic activity, the physiotherapist coaches him/her in performing a baseline measurement, setting goals, and presenting the gradual increase in a scheme.

Enabling Self-Management and Coping with Arthritic Knee Pain Through Exercise (ESCAPE-Knee Pain)

Overview

The intervention ESCAPE-knee pain has been developed by Hurley et al. [11] and aims to change the behavior of participants by challenging inappropriate beliefs about their condition and physical activity, enabling self-management and encouraging physical activity. It is based on the principles of cognitive behavioral therapy and is an integrated program, which can be delivered to either groups (of eight to ten participants) or individually. In total, ESCAPE exists of 12 sessions, held twice a week for 6 weeks. By the end of the program, participants have learnt how to utilize physical activity to self-manage their symptoms.

Content of Treatment Sessions

Each rehabilitation session starts with 15–20 min of integrated patient education, with self-management and pain-coping strategies. Sessions are interactive and include active problem solving where appropriate. Each session has different educational content and objectives. The content and aim of the education sessions are topics like exercise beliefs, determination of personal objectives and goal setting, home exercises, diet and healthy eating, drug management, pacing and activity-rest cycling, managing flares in pain, and relaxation techniques.

In the next 35–45 min, an individualized progressive exercise program is performed. The exercise specificity depends on the ability of participants and their rate of progression and therefore varies between participants and within participants over time. The complexity and intensity of the exercises are increased through mutual agreement between physiotherapists and participants. The detailed aims and content of ESCAPE have been published by Hurley et al. [11].

The Modified Arthritis Self-Management Program

Overview

The modified ASMP has been developed by Yip et al. [12] and is a combination of the existing ASMP and an exercise program. It includes six 2-h classes, once a week, with 10–15 participants, led by trained nurses.

Arthritis Self-Management Program

The Arthritis Self-Management Program has been developed by Lorig et al. [13] and is a six-session (2 h) health education program designed to help people better understand their arthritis. It is based on Bandura's concept of self-efficacy and behavior change [14]. During these six sessions, the following topics are covered: techniques to deal with problems such as pain, fatigue, social isolation, and frustration; appropriate exercises to maintain and/or improve strength, mobility, and endurance; appropriate use of medication; effective communication with family, friends, and health care providers; healthy eating; making well-informed treatment decisions; disease-related problem solving; and getting a good night's sleep.

Exercise Component

The exercise component of this program [12] consists of an action plan of three types of exercise, namely stretching exercises, walking, and Thai Chi types of movement. Before each class session, each participant is asked to set an action plan on the three exercises. During the course, the action plans are reinforced and promoted weekly. In each session, the group practices the stretching exercises together. Thai Chi exercises are taught and reinforced for half an hour in each session. To reinforce walking, a pedometer is given to the participants.

Effectiveness of Exercise Therapy Integrating Behavioral or Self-Management Mechanisms

In this paragraph, the effectiveness of interventions, which integrate exercise therapy with behavioral components and/or self-management, is described. First, the effectiveness of BGA, ESCAPE, and the modified ASMP is presented. Thereafter, the effectiveness of similar interventions is described.

Behavioral Graded Activity

Veenhof et al. and Pisters et al. [8, 15, 16] compared BGA with usual physiotherapy according to the Dutch OA guideline in 200 patients with OA of hip and/or knee. Both groups showed beneficial within-group effects in the outcome measures pain and limitations of activities, both in short and long term. In patients with knee OA, no differences between treatments were found. In patients with hip OA, significant differences in favor of BGA were found in the outcome measures pain and activity limitations, both after 3 and 9 months.

After 5 years, both interventions had similar beneficial effects on pain and limitations of activities for both patients with hip and/or knee OA. However, for patients with hip OA, BGA resulted in less joint replacement surgeries (after 5 years) compared to usual physiotherapy. Also, patients treated with BGA had more beneficial effects on the level of physical activity and adherence to exercise.

ESCAPE-Knee Pain

The effectiveness of the ESCAPE-knee pain intervention was investigated among 418 patients with chronic knee pain. Six months after completing the ESCAPE-knee intervention, participants had significantly less limitations in activity, less pain, and more improvement in psychosocial outcomes compared to usual physiotherapy [11]. Mode of delivery—individual or group treatment—did not have impact on outcome. After 12 months, the beneficial effects of ESCAPE-knee pain and usual physiotherapy were similar. However, the health care costs of ESCAPE-knee pain was lower which made ESCAPE-knee pain more cost-effective [17]. After 30 months, ESCAPE-knee pain still resulted in less activity limitations and less costs [18].

Modified ASMP Intervention

The modified ASMP intervention was compared to usual care (as prescribed by orthopedic doctor or outpatient clinic) in patients with OA of the knee. After 16 weeks, the participants of the modified ASMP intervention showed significantly more beneficial effects on pain, amount of physical activity, activity limitations, and self-efficacy compared to the control group [12]. After 12 months, significant differences were still found on the outcome measures pain and self-efficacy [19].

Further Evidence on Integrated Interventions

A systematic review has been performed on the effectiveness of combined exercise and self-management regimens in the management of lower limb OA [20]. Studies were excluded from this review if the exercise element consisted of merely advice to exercise and/or if the self-management consisted of written instruction alone and was nonparticipative. In total, ten studies were included in this review. It was concluded that these interventions reduced pain and improved activity limitations. The exercise interventions mainly consisted of a variety of lower limb strengthening, stretching, mobilizing, and balance exercises. One study included a walking program. Six interventions lasted 6–8 weeks, three interventions lasted 10–12 weeks, and one intervention continued for 18 months. Interventions were delivered to individuals or small groups, at home or in clinics or community centers. The content of the self-management component generally included advice and education on OA, healthy lifestyles (regular exercise/physical activity, healthy diet, and healthy weight) and pain-management techniques and varied in duration (from minimal instruction/education to 12 sessions). Two interventions were based on the ASMP. The self-management program was delivered by a variety of healthcare professionals including nurses, physiotherapists, and GPs. The control interventions varied from no intervention to GP care and education. In spite of the variety in interventions and the methodological flaws (such as low statistical power and short follow-up), meta-analyses showed significant beneficial effects of integrated exercise/self-management interventions on pain and activity limitations [21].

Several other studies have been performed on the effectiveness of integrated interventions, not included in the review. A chronic disease management program, using a group-based, cognitive-behavioral approach, including sessions on goal setting, pacing, symptom management, exercises and education about OA, resulted in moderate improvements in pain, activity limitations, and self-efficacy in patients with severe knee OA. Unfortunately, the results were not compared to a control group [22].

The exercise and behavior-change program Fit and Strong! was compared to the Arthritis Handbook and exercise advice in patients with knee or hip OA. Beneficial results for Fit and Strong! were found on pain and limitations of activities, self-efficacy, exercise adherence, and performance measures after 12 months [23].

Murphy et al. [24] reported the results of an Activity Strategy Training (AST), which is a structured rehabilitation program, designed to teach adaptive strategies for symptom control and engagement in physical activity and is taught by occupational therapists. The effects of AST were investigated in a pilot study involving 51 patients with knee or hip OA. In the short-term AST resulted in higher levels of physical activity compared to exercise plus health education. Although not statistically significant, participants of AST showed more improvement in pain and activity limitations. No differences were found for self-efficacy. Future studies are needed to examine larger samples and long-term effects of AST.

A pilot study was performed on the effects of an exercise-based rehabilitation program (including supervised exercises and education, coping, and self-management) in patients with hip OA. Immediately following rehabilitation, all outcome measures improved, although these improvements diminished after 6 months. There were no differences compared to usual GP care [25].

A comparison of strength training, self-management, and the combination (strength training and self-management) was made in 201 patients with early OA of the knee [26]. After 24 months, the three groups showed beneficial effects in pain and activity limitations; there were no significant differences between the groups.

Hay et al. [27] compared community physiotherapy (consisting of advice about activity and pacing and an individualized exercise program) with control (advice leaflet reinforced by telephone call) in patients with knee pain (including patients with knee OA). After 3 months, beneficial effects were found for pain and activity limitations. However, these effects disappeared in the long term.

Conclusion

In the last decade, interventions integrating behavioral strategies with exercise therapy treatments have been developed and evaluated. Despite heterogeneity of the interventions, it can be concluded that these integrated programs reduce pain and activity limitations in patients with hip and knee OA. All studies indicated beneficial effects in the short term, but the majority of studies also found improvements in the long term.

Considering the avoidance behavior of a large group of patients with OA, it is interesting whether these integrated interventions are also successful in reducing avoidance of activity behavior in this patient population. There are indeed indications that an integration of behavioral mechanisms and exercise therapy treatment has positive effects on patients' physical activity behavior. All three studies that included physical activity as outcome measure found beneficial effects on physical activity in favor of the integrated interventions [8, 12, 16, 19, 24].

An interesting question is whether integrated interventions have more beneficial results compared to exercise therapy or self-management interventions alone. Only a few studies have made such a comparison. The conclusions of these studies were diverse. Considering the BGA and ESCAPE interventions, the integrated interventions had a better outcome on activity limitations than exercise therapy. On the other hand, the integrated interventions resulted in a similar reduction of pain as exercise therapy. Moreover, Hurley et al. [21] compared the results of a meta-analysis of interventions integrating self-management within exercise therapy and the results of a meta-analysis of exercise therapy alone. These authors concluded that these types of interventions lead to similar outcomes on pain and activity limitations. However, existing studies investigating the effectiveness of integrated exercise therapy appeared to be very heterogeneous; several studies were underpowered or of low quality. To get more insight in the effectiveness of interventions integrating exercise therapy and self-management/behavioral mechanisms, high-quality studies need to be performed.

The implementation of integrated programs needs some further consideration. Some programs seem to be rather complex and time-consuming creating a barrier to implementation [21]. It is currently being explored whether interventions based on web-based applications or booklets can replace psychological counseling or self-management training. Integrated programs would become more feasible if exercise could be effectively combined with web-based applications or booklets. Cost-effectiveness studies with long-term follow-up assessments are needed to investigate which delivery mode is most effective for patients with OA.

Physiotherapists need appropriate training in order to be able to successfully implement integrated programs. They need training in basic counseling skills.

They also need to understand and accept their role as coach of the patient, providing nondirective counseling instead of directive treatment. The role as coach is quite different from the role as therapist, which is traditionally being taught to physiotherapists. Finally, physiotherapists need to have some basic understanding of psychological disorders; they need to be able to recognize these disorders and they need to know when to consult a psychologist or psychiatrist [28]. Developing appropriate training in the skills required for integrated programs is a major future challenge.

References

1. Pisters MF, Veenhof C, van Meeteren NLU, Ostelo RW, de Bakker DH, Schellevis FG et al (2007) Long-term effectiveness of exercise therapy in patients with osteoarthritis of hip or knee: a systematic review. Arthritis Rheum 57(7):1245–1253
2. Pisters MF, Veenhof C, van Dijk GM, Heymans MW, Twisk JW, Dekker J (2012) The course of limitations in activities over five years in patients with knee and hip osteoarthritis with moderate functional limitations: risk factors for future functional decline. Osteoarthritis Cartilage 20(6):503–510
3. Dziedzic KS, Hill JC, Porcheret M, Croft PR (2009) New models for primary care are needed for osteoarthritis. Phys Ther 89(12):1371–1378
4. Keefe FJ, Somers TJ, Martire LM (2008) Psychologic interventions and lifestyle modifications for arthritis pain management. Rheum Dis Clin North Am 34(2):351–368
5. NICE 2008 (2012) Osteoarthritis: the care and management of osteoarthritis in adults. Ref type: Internet communication
6. Zhang W, Moskowitz RW, Nuki G, Abramson S, Altman RD, Arden N et al (2008) OARSI recommendations for the management of hip and knee osteoarthritis, part II: OARSI evidence-based, expert consensus guidelines. Osteoarthritis Cartilage 16(2):137–162
7. Buszewicz M, Rait G, Griffin M, Nazareth I, Patel A, Atkinson A et al (2006) Self management of arthritis in primary care: randomised controlled trial. BMJ 333(7574):879
8. Veenhof C (2006) Effectiveness of behavioral graded activity in patients with osteoarthritis of the hip and/or knee: a randomized clinical trial. Arthritis Rheum 55(6):925–934
9. Fordyce WE, Fowler RS, Lehmann JF, Delateur BJ, Sand PL, Trieschmann RB (1973) Operant conditioning in the treatment of chronic pain. Arch Phys Med Rehabil 54:339–408
10. Lindstrom I, Ohlund C, Eek C, Wallin L, Peterson LE, Fordyce WE et al (1992) The effect of graded activity on patients with subacute low back pain: a randomized prospective clinical study with an operant-conditioning behavioral approach. Phys Ther 72(4):279–290
11. Hurley MV, Walsh NE, Mitchell HL, Pimm TJ, Patel A, Williamson E et al (2007) Clinical effectiveness of a rehabilitation program integrating exercise, self-management, and active coping strategies for chronic knee pain: a cluster randomized trial. Arthritis Rheum 57(7):1211–1219
12. Yip YB (2007) Effects of a self-management arthritis programme with an added exercise component for osteoarthritic knee: randomized controlled trial. J Adv Nurs 59(1):20–28
13. Lorig KR, Mazonson PD, Holman HR (1993) Evidence suggesting that health education for self-management in patients with chronic arthritis has sustained health benefits while reducing health care costs. Arthritis Rheum 36(4):439–446
14. Bandura A (1986) Social foundation of thought and action: a social cognitive theory. Prestice-Hall, Englewood Cliffs, NJ
15. Pisters MF, Veenhof C, de Bakker DH, Schellevis FG, Dekker J (2010) Long-term effectiveness of exercise therapy in patients with osteoarthritis of the hip or knee: a randomized

controlled trial comparing two different physiotherapy interventions. Osteoarthritis Cartilage 18(8):1019–1026

16. Pisters MF, Veenhof C, de Bakker DH, Schellevis FG, Dekker J (2010) Behavioural graded activity results in better exercise adherence and more physical activity than usual care in people with osteoarthritis: a cluster-randomised trial. J Physiother 56(1):41–47
17. Jessep SA, Walsh NE, Ratcliffe J, Hurley MV (2009 Jun) Long-term clinical benefits and costs of an integrated rehabilitation programme compared with outpatient physiotherapy for chronic knee pain. Physiotherapy 95(2):94–102
18. Hurley MV, Walsh NE, Mitchell H, Nicholas J, Patel A (2012) Long-term outcomes and costs of an integrated rehabilitation program for chronic knee pain: a pragmatic, cluster randomized, controlled trial. Arthritis Care Res (Hoboken) 64(2):238–247
19. Yip YB, Sit JW, Wong DY, Chong SY, Chung LH (2008) A 1-year follow-up of an experimental study of a self-management arthritis programme with an added exercise component of clients with osteoarthritis of the knee. Psychol Health Med 13(4):402–414
20. Walsh NE, Mitchell HL, Reeves BC, Hurley MV (2006) Integrated exercise and self-management programmes in osteoarthritis of the hip and knee: a systematic review of effectiveness. Phys Ther Rev 11:289–297
21. Hurley MV, Walsh NE (2009) Effectiveness and clinical applicability of integrated rehabilitation programs for knee osteoarthritis. Curr Opin Rheumatol 21(2):171–176
22. Lamb SE, Toye F, Barker KL (2008) Chronic disease management programme in people with severe knee osteoarthritis: efficacy and moderators of response. Clin Rehabil 22(2):169–178
23. Hughes SL, Seymour RB, Campbell RT, Huber G, Pollak N, Sharma L et al (2006) Long-term impact of fit and strong! On older adults with osteoarthritis. Gerontologist 46(6):801–814
24. Murphy SL, Strasburg DM, Lyden AK, Smith DM, Koliba JF, Dadabhoy DP et al (2008) Effects of activity strategy training on pain and physical activity in older adults with knee or hip osteoarthritis: a pilot study. Arthritis Rheum 59(10):1480–1487
25. Bearne LM, Walsh NE, Jessep S, Hurley MV (2011) Feasibility of an exercise-based rehabilitation programme for chronic hip pain. Musculoskeletal Care. doi:10.1002/msc.209
26. McKnight PE, Kasle S, Going S, Villanueva I, Cornett M, Farr J et al (2010) A comparison of strength training, self-management, and the combination for early osteoarthritis of the knee. Arthritis Care Res (Hoboken) 62(1):45–53
27. Hay EM, Foster NE, Thomas E, Peat G, Phelan M, Yates HE et al (2006) Effectiveness of community physiotherapy and enhanced pharmacy review for knee pain in people aged over 55 presenting to primary care: pragmatic randomised trial. BMJ 333(7576):995
28. Dekker J, van der Valk RWA, Verhaak PFM (1995) Psychosocial complaints and physical therapy. Physiother Theory Pract 11:175–186

Chapter 10
Comorbidity, Obesity, and Exercise Therapy in Patients with Knee and Hip Osteoarthritis

Mariëtte de Rooij, Willem F. Lems, Marike van der Leeden, and Joost Dekker

Comorbidity in OA

Comorbidity is highly prevalent in patients with knee and hip osteoarthritis (OA) [1]. Feinstein defined comorbidity as "any distinct additional clinical entity that has existed or that may occur during the clinical course of a patient who has the index disease (i.e. *osteoarthritis*; italics added) under study." Studies have reported comorbidity rates of 68–85 % [2–5]. Comorbidities that often occur next to OA are cardiac diseases, hypertension, respiratory diseases, diseases of eye, ear, nose, throat and larynx, urogenital diseases, overweight/obesity, low back pain, and endocrine and metabolic diseases [1, 2, 5, 6]. OA patients frequently suffer several comorbidities [4].

Comorbidity in patients with knee and hip OA is associated with more limitations in daily activities, e.g., walking, stair climbing, and rising up from of a chair. A limited number of studies have addressed the impact of comorbidities on activity limitations and pain. Van Reeuwijk et al. [7] reported that several categories of comorbidity are associated with more activity limitations: musculoskeletal disorders (chronic low back pain or hernia, arthritis of hands or feet, and other rheumatic diseases); non-musculoskeletal disorders (diabetes and chronic cystitis); sensory impairments (dizziness in combination with falling, and visual and hearing impairments); and finally overweight and obesity. Cardiac diseases

M. de Rooij • M. van der Leeden
Amsterdam Rehabilitation Research Center | Reade, Amsterdam, The Netherlands

W.F. Lems
Department of Rheumatology, VU University Medical Center, Amsterdam, The Netherlands

J. Dekker (✉)
Department of Rehabilitation Medicine, VU University Medical Center, PO Box 7057, 1007 MB Amsterdam, The Netherlands

Department of Psychiatry, VU University Medical Center, Amsterdam, The Netherlands
e-mail: j.dekker@vumc.nl

J. Dekker (ed.), *Exercise and Physical Functioning in Osteoarthritis: Medical, Neuromuscular and Behavioral Perspectives*, Springer Briefs in Specialty Topics in Behavioral Medicine, DOI 10.1007/978-1-4614-7215-5_10, © The Author(s) 2014

[2, 5, 8] and depression [9] are also associated with more activity limitations. Comorbidities that are associated with pain include musculoskeletal disorders (arthritis of the hands or feet, and other rheumatic diseases) and diabetes [7]. It is also known that patients with generalized OA report more pain than patients with hip or knee OA alone [10].

Comorbidity and Exercise

Exercise therapy is one of the key recommendations in current guidelines for the management of OA [11–16]. Exercise therapy is effective in relieving pain and improving daily functioning in patients with knee OA [17, 18] and most likely also for hip OA [19]. For patients with knee or hip OA, regular exercise therapy consist of exercises aimed at strengthening lower-limb muscles, improving aerobic capacity, range of knee joint motion (ROM), joint stability, and training of daily activities like walking, stair climbing, and transfers. An extensive description of training modalities in patients with OA is given elsewhere in this volume (see Chap. 7).

The presence of comorbidity may limit the application of exercise therapy. In fact, in clinical practice patients with (severe) comorbidity are often not referred for exercise therapy, or drop out at an early stage of treatment and/or are treated inadequately. Therapists often reduce the intensity of the treatment to a level where it is unlikely to be effective, as protocols and guidelines do not offer advice concerning comorbidity-associated adaptations [11–16].

When comorbidity is present, it may be necessary to adapt the OA exercise program in order to avoid serious adverse events and to increase the effectiveness of exercise. In some cases, exercise may be fully contraindicated. For example, an absolute contraindication for exercise therapy is a resting systolic blood pressure of ≥200 mmHg or a diastolic blood pressure of ≥115 mmHg [20]. In other cases, exercise is possible, if exercise is tailored to the condition of the patient. For example, in patients with OA and COPD, interval training may be indicated instead of endurance training because of dyspnea.

A few studies have evaluated the effects of exercise in patients with OA and comorbidity. Two studies [21, 22] reported on predictors of the outcome of exercise, concluding that comorbidity is related to a poor treatment outcome. In contrast, in the FAST study, secondary analyses indicated that the presence of comorbidity did not substantially affect the outcome of the exercise program on physical performance [23]. However, as in many other studies, patients with severe comorbid diseases were excluded from participation in that study.

Restrictions and Contraindications

Our research group has identified contraindications and restrictions for exercise in common comorbidities in OA [24]. *Contraindications* are defined as conditions fully precluding the application of exercise therapy: the patient should be excluded from exercise therapy. For example, pneumonia or exceptional loss of bodyweight is an absolute contraindication for exercise in patients with COPD. *Restrictions* are defined as conditions limiting the application of exercise therapy, necessitating adaptations to the therapeutic protocol. For example, in patients with chronic heart failure, breathlessness and fatigue disproportional to the level of exertion should be avoided by adapting the training intensity, because of the risk of cardiac decompensation [25].

We have searched the literature for restrictions and contraindications for exercise therapy in highly prevalent comorbidities in OA. It was found that cardiac diseases, hypertension, type 2 diabetes, and COPD are associated with restrictions resulting mainly from physiological impairments. This group of comorbidities has a high risk of exercise-related adverse events. For example, in patients with coronary heart disease with unstable angina patient safety during exercise therapy cannot always be guaranteed, resulting in an absolute contraindication for exercise therapy. A restriction to exercise consists in patients with diabetes because of an increased risk of wounds due to sensibility loss of the feet; closed kinematic chain exercises may be contraindicated; open kinematic chain exercises may be indicated to relieve stress and pressure on the feet. Within this group of comorbidities, the intensity of training needs to be adapted to allow safe and effective exercise. With appropriate adaptations, it is likely that patient safety can be ensured and adverse events prevented.

Obesity is associated with restrictions resulting from physiological and psychological impairments and behavioral barriers. For example, a physiological restriction in these patients is a poor thermoregulation during exertion. During warmer climatic conditions, the exercise program should be adapted by reducing the training intensity.

Low back pain, chronic pain syndromes, and depression are associated mainly with psychological and behavioral restrictions to exercise therapy. This group of comorbidities has a low risk of adverse events; restrictions to OA exercise are more related to psychological or behavioral barriers, e.g., avoidance of exercise. Within this group of comorbidities, adaptations should be made by using a time-contingent approach, which focuses on improvement of activities in daily life and not on pain relief.

Visual and hearing impairments result predominantly in environmental restrictions to exercise. In this group of comorbidities, adaptations should be made by changes in equipment, conditions (e.g., lighting), or treatment location.

Adaptations in Exercise Therapy in Patients with Knee OA and Comorbidity

OA exercise can be tailored to the comorbidity by adapting duration, frequency, intensity, or type (content) of the exercise therapy. The exact adaptation of exercise depends on the nature and severity of the comorbidity and the restrictions for exercise therapy, as identified by the physical therapist in the diagnostic phase.

We have developed comorbidity-adapted exercise protocols for comorbidities that are highly prevalent in OA and have impact on pain and daily functioning: cardiac diseases, hypertension, diabetes type 2, obesity, chronic obstructive pulmonary disease (COPD), depression, chronic pain, low back pain, and visual or hearing impairments.

Guidelines on exercise therapy in cardiac diseases [26, 27], diabetes [28], and COPD [29], nonspecific low back pain [30] have been issued. These guidelines describe the preferred approach toward the physiotherapeutic diagnosis and treatment (i.e., exercise). The principles described in these guidelines have been incorporated into the comorbidity-adapted exercise protocols for OA. For example, in patients with OA and cardiac diseases, the aerobic training intensity can be set by using heart frequency or rate of perceived exertion (scale 6–20).

In the protocol on exercise in OA patients with comorbidity, adaptations are made in the diagnostic and intervention phase of exercise therapy.

The Diagnostic Phase. The diagnostic phase consists of anamnesis, physical examination, and the establishment of treatment goals and determination of the treatment strategy. During anamnesis, OA-related problems and comorbidity-related restrictions and contraindications for exercise therapy are identified. A clinical decision is made whether physical examination is possible or whether the referring physician has to be consulted first, because of contraindications for physical examination or the need for additional medical information. With respect to the latter, test results of an exercise symptom limited test may be required for patients with heart failure to establish the training intensity.

If there are no contraindications for physical examination, an examination is performed concerning impairments and activity limitations related to both OA and comorbidity. For example, it may be needed to test the sensibility of the feet in patients with diabetes type 2. Subsequently, a clinical decision is made whether there are contraindications or restrictions to exercise therapy. If there are contraindications for exercise, the patient is referred back to the specialist. If there are restrictions related to comorbidity, a comorbidity-adapted program is indicated. In this phase, the therapist may also consider whether consultation of other disciplines is indicated, e.g., a dietician, psychologist, or occupational therapist. For example, this might be a consultation of a dietician for patients with overweight or obesity.

Intervention Phase. In the intervention phase, exercise programs are tailored to the comorbidity by adapting duration, frequency, intensity, and type of exercise therapy. The exact adaptation depends on the restrictions for exercise therapy identified by the therapist in the diagnostic phase. Comorbidity may necessitate several different or even contradictory adaptations in exercises. The inherent variation and complexity of comorbidities make tailoring of treatment a requirement, based on clinical reasoning. The specific options for adaptations to OA exercises are listed in the protocol and are summarized below.

Comorbidities like cardiac disease, hypertension, type 2 diabetes, and COPD are mostly associated with restrictions resulting from exercise-related physiological impairments. Within this group of comorbidities, adaptations are made to OA exercise programs by reducing intensity or duration of aerobic, strengthening, and/or functional exercises. Our protocol describes how the individual maximum training capacity of the patient can be reached in patients with cardiac disease, hypertension, diabetes, or COPD.

In patients with obesity and high levels of pain in the knees or hips, adaptations in weight-bearing exercises may be indicated. Also, reduced-intensity aerobic exercises may be indicated in this population because of shortness of breath as a result of deconditioning. The reduction of exercise intensity, coupled with adequate hydration during exercise, is of great importance in warmer climatic conditions because of impaired thermoregulation. Finally, the provision of information about the importance of weight reduction, and stimulation herein, are important (possibly under supervision of a dietician).

Nonspecific low back pain, chronic pain syndromes, and depression are associated with psychological and behavioral restrictions to exercise therapy. Within this group of comorbidities, a behavioral approach is indicated. In a time-contingent manner, the amount of physical activity can be gradually increased combined with a gradual increase in the level of regular OA exercise, e.g., strengthening exercises of the lower limbs. In addition, patients receive education about pain and coaching on how to cope with stress and fear of movement. Further, a positive attitude toward physical activities is encouraged.

Visual and hearing impairments result predominantly in environmental restrictions to exercise. Within these comorbidities, environmental restrictions lead to adaptations in training equipment, treatment location, training conditions (e.g., lighting), and changes in the way patients are handled, e.g., using more manual guidance, and checking whether or not the patient has understood the information.

Our comorbid-adapted protocols were evaluated in a pilot study on patients with knee OA and comorbidity. The protocol appeared to be useful in clinical decision making for the diagnostic and treatment phase in patients with knee OA patients with comorbid diseases; therapists indicated that the protocol helped them to tailor the exercise program to the individual capacity of the patient. No adverse events occurred. Quantitative evaluation of the treatment outcome showed improvements of activity limitations and pain. However, further studies are needed to confirm and expand our findings.

Exercise Therapy in Patients with OA and Overweight or Obesity

Several studies have evaluated the effectiveness of weight loss and physical activity in patients with knee OA and overweight. Weight reduction using a diet has been proven to be effective and is recommended in national and international guidelines in knee OA patients [31, 32]. In patients with hip OA, this recommendation is based on expert opinion, as no studies are yet available. In a systematic review [33], it is concluded that weight loss results in decreased pain and improved function, most notably when a diet is combined with physical exercise [34, 35]. In this review, the authors also suggest that weight loss of >5 % within a 20-week period is related to symptomatic relief. Weight loss under supervision of a dietician seems to be more effective than just giving dietary advice [36].

Conclusion

Comorbidity is highly prevalent and is associated with more activity limitations and pain in patients with knee or hip OA. We have developed comorbidity-adapted exercise protocols, which support the therapist in tailoring the OA exercise program to the individual capacity of the patient. We are currently evaluating the impact of these protocols on activity limitations and pain in OA patients with comorbidity.

References

1. Schellevis FG, van der Velden J, van de Lisdonk E, van Eijk JT, van Weel C (1993) Comorbidity of chronic diseases in general practice. J Clin Epidemiol 46(5):469–473
2. Caporali R, Cimmino MA, Sarzi-Puttini P, Scarpa R, Parazzini F, Zaninelli A et al (2005) Comorbid conditions in the AMICA study patients: effects on the quality of life and drug prescriptions by general practitioners and specialists. Semin Arthritis Rheum 35(1 Suppl 1): 31–37
3. Juhakoski R, Tenhonen S, Anttonen T, Kauppinen T, Arokoski JP (2008) Factors affecting self-reported pain and physical function in patients with hip osteoarthritis. Arch Phys Med Rehabil 89(6):1066–1073
4. Tuominen U, Blom M, Hirvonen J, Seitsalo S, Lehto M, Paavolainen P et al (2007) The effect of co-morbidities on health-related quality of life in patients placed on the waiting list for total joint replacement. Health Qual Life Outcomes 5:16
5. van Dijk GM, Veenhof C, Schellevis F, Hulsmans H, Bakker JP, Arwert H et al (2008) Comorbidity, limitations in activities and pain in patients with osteoarthritis of the hip or knee. BMC Musculoskelet Disord 9:95
6. Kadam UT, Jordan K, Croft PR (2004) Clinical comorbidity in patients with osteoarthritis: a case-control study of general practice consulters in England and Wales. Ann Rheum Dis 63(4):408–414
7. Reeuwijk KG, de Rooij M, van Dijk GM, Veenhof C, Steultjens MP, Dekker J (2010) Osteoarthritis of the hip or knee: which coexisting disorders are disabling? Clin Rheumatol 29(7):739–747
8. Ettinger WH, Davis MA, Neuhaus JM, Mallon KP (1994) Long-term physical functioning in persons with knee osteoarthritis from NHANES. I: effects of comorbid medical conditions. J Clin Epidemiol 47(7):809–815
9. Dunlop DD, Semanik P, Song J, Manheim LM, Shih V, Chang RW (2005) Risk factors for functional decline in older adults with arthritis. Arthritis Rheum 52(4):1274–1282
10. Cimmino MA, Sarzi-Puttini P, Scarpa R, Caporali R, Parazzini F, Zaninelli A et al (2005) Clinical presentation of osteoarthritis in general practice: determinants of pain in Italian patients in the AMICA study. Semin Arthritis Rheum 35(1 Suppl 1):17–23

11. American College of Rheumatology Subcommittee on Osteoarthritis Guidelines (2000) Recommendations for the medical management of osteoarthritis of the hip and knee: 2000 update. Arthritis Rheum 43(9):1905–1915
12. Jordan KM, Arden NK, Doherty M, Bannwarth B, Bijlsma JW, Dieppe P et al (2003) EULAR recommendations 2003: an evidence based approach to the management of knee osteoarthritis: report of a Task Force of the Standing Committee for International Clinical Studies Including Therapeutic Trials (ESCISIT). Ann Rheum Dis 62(12):1145–1155
13. Conaghan PG, Dickson J, Grant RL (2008) Care and management of osteoarthritis in adults: summary of NICE guidance. BMJ 336(7642):502–503
14. Zhang W, Doherty M, Arden N, Bannwarth B, Bijlsma J, Gunther KP et al (2005) EULAR evidence based recommendations for the management of hip osteoarthritis: report of a task force of the EULAR Standing Committee for International Clinical Studies Including Therapeutics (ESCISIT). Ann Rheum Dis 64(5):669–681
15. Zhang W, Moskowitz RW, Nuki G, Abramson S, Altman RD, Arden N et al (2008) OARSI recommendations for the management of hip and knee osteoarthritis, part II: OARSI evidence-based, expert consensus guidelines. Osteoarthritis Cartilage 16(2):137–162
16. Zhang W, Moskowitz RW, Nuki G, Abramson S, Altman RD, Arden N et al (2007) OARSI recommendations for the management of hip and knee osteoarthritis, part I: critical appraisal of existing treatment guidelines and systematic review of current research evidence. Osteoarthritis Cartilage 15(9):981–1000
17. van Baar ME, Assendelft WJ, Dekker J, Oostendorp RA, Bijlsma JW (1999) Effectiveness of exercise therapy in patients with osteoarthritis of the hip or knee: a systematic review of randomized clinical trials. Arthritis Rheum 42(7):1361–1369
18. Smidt N, de Vet HC, Bouter LM, Dekker J, Arendzen JH, de Bie RA et al (2005) Effectiveness of exercise therapy: a best-evidence summary of systematic reviews. Aust J Physiother 51(2):71–85
19. Fransen M, McConnell S, Hernandez-Molina G, Reichenbach S (2009) Exercise for osteoarthritis of the hip. Cochrane Database Syst Rev 3:CD007912
20. Gordon NF (2003) Hypertension. In: Durstine JL, Moore GE (eds) ACSM's exercise management for persons with chronic diseases and disabilities. Human Kinetics, Champaign, IL, pp 76–80
21. Jansen MJ, Hendriks EJ, Oostendorp RA, Dekker J, de Bie RA (2010) Quality indicators indicate good adherence to the clinical practice guideline on "Osteoarthritis of the hip and knee" and few prognostic factors influence outcome indicators: a prospective cohort study. Eur J Phys Rehabil Med 46(3):337–345
22. Tamari K (2010) Baseline comorbidity associated with the short-term effects of exercise intervention on quality of life in the Japanese older population: an observational study. Arch Phys Med Rehabil 91(9):1363–1369
23. Mangani I, Cesari M, Kritchevsky SB, Maraldi C, Carter CS, Atkinson HH et al (2006) Physical exercise and comorbidity. Results from the Fitness and Arthritis in Seniors Trial (FAST). Aging Clin Exp Res 18(5):374–380
24. de Rooij M, Steultjens MPM, Avezaat E, Häkkinen A, Klaver R, van der Leeden M et al (2013) Restrictions and contraindications for exercise therapy in patients with hip and knee osteoarthritis and comorbidity. Phys Ther Rev 18(2):101–111
25. Coats AJ (2001) Exercise and heart failure. Cardiol Clin 19(3):517–524, xii–xiii
26. Revalidatie commissie van de Nederlandse vereniging voor cardiologie en de Nederlandse Hartstichting (2004) Richtlijn Hartrevalidatie 2004. Nederlandse Harstichting, Den Haag
27. Vogels EMHM, Bertram RJJ, Graus JJJ, Hendriks HJM, van Hulst R, Hulzebos HJ et al (2005) Cardiac rehabilitation guideline, The Royal Dutch Society for Physical Therapy (KNGF). KNGF, Amersfoort
28. Werkgroep Sport en Bewegen van de Nederlandse Diabetes Federatie (2000) Sport en bewegen bij diabetes mellitus. Leusden

29. Gosselink R, Langer D, Burton C, Probst V, Hendriks HJM, van der Schans CP et al (2008) Chronic obstructive pulmonary disease guideline, The Royal Dutch Society for Physical Therapy (KNGF). KNGF, Amersfoort
30. Bekkering GE, Hendriks HJM, Koes BW, Oostendorp RAB, Ostelo RWJG, Thomassen J et al (2001) Low back pain guideline, The Royal Dutch Society for Physical Therapy (KNGF). KNGF, Amersfoort
31. Peter WFH, Jansen MJ, Bloo H, Dekker-Bakker LMMC, Dilling RG, Hilberdink WKH et al (2010) Osteoarthritis of the hip and knee guideline, The Royal Dutch Society for Physical Therapy (KNGF). KNGF, Amersfoort
32. Zhang W, Nuki G, Moskowitz RW, Abramson S, Altman RD, Arden NK et al (2010) OARSI recommendations for the management of hip and knee osteoarthritis: part III: changes in evidence following systematic cumulative update of research published through January 2009. Osteoarthritis Cartilage 18(4):476–499
33. Christensen R, Bartels EM, Astrup A, Bliddal H (2007) Effect of weight reduction in obese patients diagnosed with knee osteoarthritis: a systematic review and meta-analysis. Ann Rheum Dis 66(4):433–439
34. Messier SP, Gutekunst DJ, Davis C, DeVita P (2005) Weight loss reduces knee-joint loads in overweight and obese older adults with knee osteoarthritis. Arthritis Rheum 52(7):2026–2032
35. Brosseau L, Wells GA, Tugwell P, Egan M, Dubouloz CJ, Casimiro L et al (2011) Ottawa Panel evidence-based clinical practice guidelines for the management of osteoarthritis in adults who are obese or overweight. Phys Ther 91(6):843–861
36. Christensen R, Astrup A, Bliddal H (2005) Weight loss: the treatment of choice for knee osteoarthritis? A randomized trial. Osteoarthritis Cartilage 13(1):20–27

Chapter 11
Summary and Future Directions

Joost Dekker

Summary

Epidemiology and Therapeutic Options

Osteoarthritis (OA) is a major public health problem, with ~16 % and ~9 % of the adult population older than 45 years suffering from symptomatic OA of the knee and hip, respectively. OA is major cause of pain and activity limitations. Therapeutic options include nonpharmacological, pharmacological, and surgical interventions. Nonpharmacological interventions are of great importance, since drugs that slow disease progression are not available. Furthermore, pharmacological therapy frequently leads to side effects, while surgical intervention is being reserved for end-stage OA. This makes exercise therapy stand out as one of the major nonpharmacological interventions. Exercise therapy is advised in all major OA-treatment guidelines.

Functional Decline: Risk Factors and Explanatory Mechanisms

The progression of pain and activity limitations in OA is slow but highly variable. The progression varies: some patients show functional decline, other patients are stable, while still other patients seem to improve.

J. Dekker (✉)
Department of Rehabilitation Medicine, VU University Medical Center, PO Box 7057, 1007 MB Amsterdam, The Netherlands

Department of Psychiatry, VU University Medical Center, Amsterdam, The Netherlands
e-mail: j.dekker@vumc.nl

J. Dekker (ed.), *Exercise and Physical Functioning in Osteoarthritis: Medical, Neuromuscular and Behavioral Perspectives*, Springer Briefs in Specialty Topics in Behavioral Medicine, DOI 10.1007/978-1-4614-7215-5_11, © The Author(s) 2014

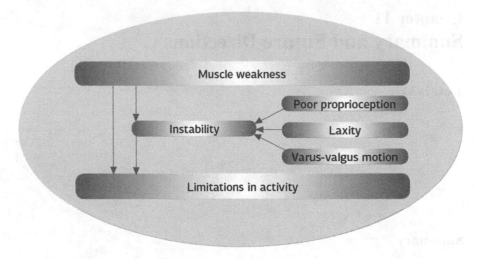

Fig. 11.1 Neuromuscular factors and activity limitations

Because of this variability, identification of risk factors for functional decline is of utmost importance. Risk factors for functional decline include impairments of body functions (pain, muscle weakness, proprioceptive inaccuracy, joint laxity, joint instability, impaired range of joint motion, and overweight), comorbidity, personal factors (age, intoxications, health behavior, coping, self-efficacy, and psychological distress), and environmental factors (social support). The predictive value of impairments of body structures (degeneration of cartilage and bone) is not clear.

The neuromuscular model aims to explain the impact of some of these neuromuscular factors risk factors (see Fig. 11.1). Muscle weakness is a crucial factor in the explanation of activity limitations in OA. Muscle weakness is thought to have a direct impact on activity limitations. Muscle weakness may also have an indirect impact on the performance of activities, through instability of the knee joint. Poor proprioception, joint laxity, and varus–valgus motion of the knee joint during walking may interact with muscle weakness, leading to joint instability and thereby activity limitations. Several studies support the validity of the neuromuscular model.

The avoidance model aims to explain the impact of psychological factors on functional decline, in particular the impact of psychological distress (anxious or depressive mood, and fatigue; see Fig. 11.2). OA patients tend to avoid activity, as physical activity causes pain. In the short term, avoidance of activity may have the desired effect of less pain. However, in the longer term, inactivity results in muscle weakness and activity limitations. Psychological distress is hypothesized to strengthen the tendency to avoid activity, thereby inducing more activity limitations. Findings from several studies indicate that the avoidance model offers a valid explanation of the impact of psychological distress on activity limitations.

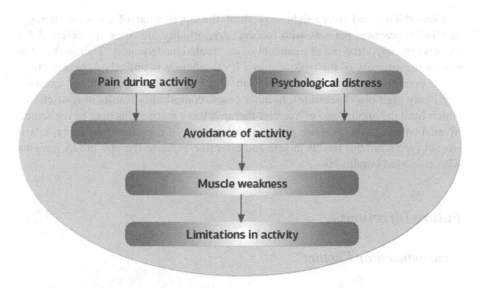

Fig. 11.2 Avoidance and activity limitations

Exercise Therapy

Exercise therapy includes exercises aiming at improvement of muscle strength, aerobic capacity, flexibility, and daily activities. Exercises can be performed under supervision (individually or in a group) or not-supervised at home. In knee OA, exercise therapy has been found to relieve pain and to reduce activity limitations. In hip OA, exercise therapy is likely to be effective, although limited evidence is available.

Although clearly effective, the effect size of exercise therapy is small to moderate. Neuromuscular exercise therapy aims to improve the outcome by addressing neuromuscular factors, other than muscle weakness. Neuromuscular exercise targets factors, such as poor proprioception, laxity, and uncontrolled motion of the knee, aiming at improved neuromuscular control. Modalities of neuromuscular exercise include agility, balance, and pertubation training. Neuromuscular exercise seems to be effective in reducing pain and activity limitations. The additional effect of exercises targeting neuromuscular mechanisms over traditional muscle strengthening programs has not been demonstrated yet.

Exercise therapy combined with psychological interventions aims at improved outcome by targeting psychological distress, cognitive factors, or improving self-management. These psychological factors are hypothesized to contribute to functional decline. Interventions combining psychological strategies with exercise therapy reduce pain and activity limitations in patients with hip and knee OA. The combined interventions seem to result in similar reductions of pain and activity limitations as regular exercise therapy. Given the limitations of existing studies, further research on combined interventions is indicated.

Comorbidity and overweight may limit the application of exercise therapy. In clinical practice, patients with (severe) comorbidity are often not referred for exercise therapy, drop out of treatment or are treated inadequately. Therapists often reduce the intensity of the treatment to a level where it is unlikely to be effective. Some comorbid conditions constitute an absolute contraindication for exercise (e.g., very high blood pressure). In other cases, comorbidity results in restrictions, which limit the application of exercise therapy; these restrictions may be overcome by adaptations to the exercise protocol. Adaptation of duration, frequency, intensity, or type (content) results in safe and effective exercise therapy in OA patients with comorbid conditions.

Future Directions

Neuromuscular Factors

In the neuromuscular model, muscle weakness is regarded the central determinant of activity limitations. Substantial evidence from cross-sectional studies supports this hypothesis. Surprisingly, little evidence from longitudinal studies on the role of muscle strength is available. There is a strong need for longitudinal studies in this area. In addition, more detailed knowledge on muscle strength and function in relation to activities in OA is needed; for example, which muscles are affected in OA, and how much strength is needed to perform activities? Furthermore, knowledge is needed on determinants of muscle weakness; for example, we have recently found an association between low-grade inflammation and muscle weakness in OA [1]. This finding opens interesting perspectives on inflammation as a potential factor in muscle weakness in OA.

Instability of the knee seems a major determinant of activity limitations. This conclusion is based on cross-sectional studies, indicating the need for longitudinal studies in this area as well. Even more importantly, current measurements of instability rely almost exclusively on self-report. Measures not relying on self-report would obviously contribute strongly to scientific progress in this area.

Avoidance

Substantial evidence supports the avoidance model as an explanation of the impact of psychological distress on activity limitations in knee OA; each of the steps in the model (i.e., the interrelationships between components of the model) is supported by scientific research. The cross-sectional nature of most studies is a major limitation, however. Cross-sectional studies do not allow causal interpretations. To further justify the causal claims of the avoidance model, evidence from longitudinal studies is required. Some evidence from longitudinal studies does support the avoidance model, which is encouraging. Longitudinal research on the interrelationships between components of the model is clearly a crucial next step in the validation process of the avoidance model.

Another major comment concerns the explanatory power of the avoidance model. The model explains part of the variance in activity limitations in knee OA. This indicates that there must be other pathways than those hypothesized in the avoidance model. Some of these pathways may involve the avoidance model. For example, low self-efficacy is associated with a higher level of limitations in activity; low self-efficacy may strengthen the tendency to avoid activity, which leads to a higher level of limitations in activity. Other psychological pathways, not involving avoidance of activity, may exist as well. Future research could explore these alternative pathways explaining limitations inactivity.

Finally, the avoidance model concerns limitations in activity in knee OA. Whether the avoidance model is a valid explanation of limitations in activity in hip OA is largely unknown. Future research could focus on the validity of the avoidance model in hip OA.

Exercise Therapy

Better understanding of neuromuscular factors, behavioral factors, and comorbidity may contribute to the development of more effective exercise therapy. Knowledge on the causes of activity limitations in OA may be used to develop exercise therapy targeting specific neuromuscular, behavioral, or comorbidity-related factors. This strategy has been shown productive; exercise programs focusing on specific neuromuscular, behavioral, or comorbidity-related factors have been developed. The effectiveness of these programs has been demonstrated. However, the superiority of these programs over traditional exercise therapy is less clear. This observation points to the need to refine the theoretical explanations of activity limitations; the need to empirically test these explanations and adapt theoretical models based on the empirical results; and the need to derive even more specific exercise programs from these improved theoretical models.

Novel approaches toward exercise therapy are indicated as well. For example, the combination of optimized pain medication with exercise therapy might be indicated in some patients. High levels of pain preclude exercise and physical activity in some patients; in these patients, pain medication may have to be optimized before patients are able to exercise. Safety and effectiveness of this approach needs to be investigated.

Finally, subgroups (phenotypes) of knee OA patients with various patterns of activity limitations and factors contributing to activity limitations have been observed [2]. It is very likely that exercise therapy needs to be tailored to characteristics of various subgroups of OA patients.

References

1. Sanchez-Ramirez DC, van der Leeden M, van der Esch M, Gerritsen M, Roorda LD, Verschueren S, van Dieën J, Dekker J, Lems WF (2013) Associations of serum C-reactive protein and erythrocyte sedimentation rate with muscle strength in patients with knee osteoarthritis. Rheumatology 52(4):727–732
2. Knoop J, van der Leeden M, Thorstensson CA et al (2011) Identification of phenotypes with different clinical outcomes in knee osteoarthritis: data from the Osteoarthritis Initiative. Arthritis Care Res 63(11):1535–1542